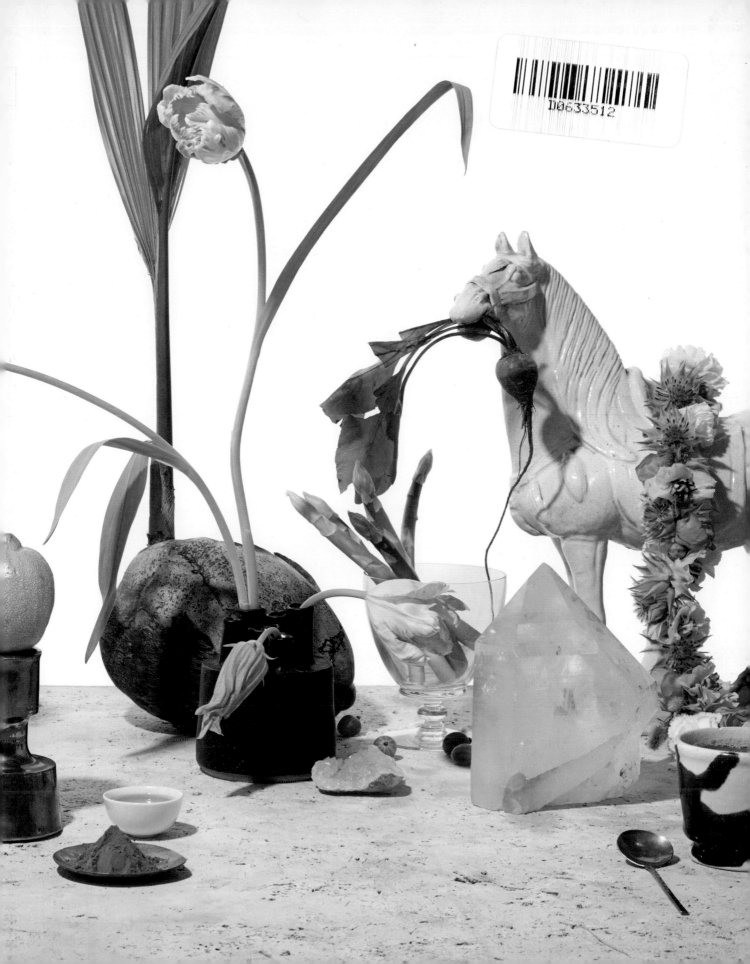

HIGH
VIBRATIONAL
BEAUTY

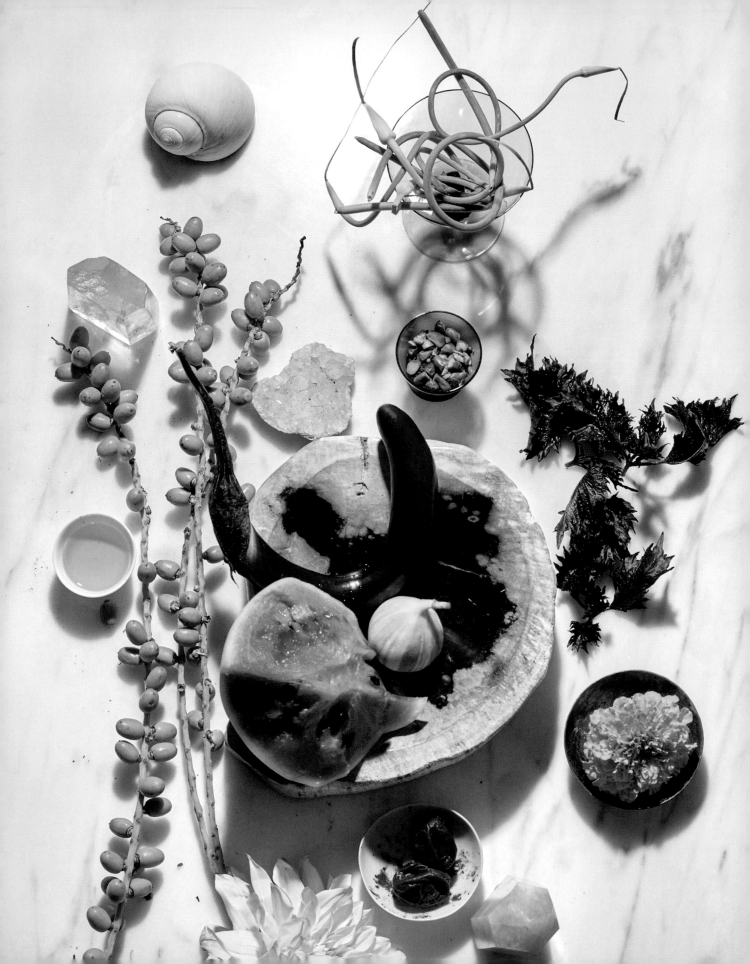

HIGH VIBRATIONAL BEAUTY

RECIPES AND RITUALS FOR RADICAL SELF CARE

KERRILYNN PAMER & CINDY DIPRIMA MORISSE

FOUNDERS OF CAP BEAUTY

RODALE.

RODALE *wellness*

Live happy. Be healthy. Get inspired.

Sign up today to get exclusive access to our authors, exclusive bonuses, and the most authoritative, useful, and cutting-edge information on health, wellness, fitness, and living your life to the fullest.

Visit us online at RodaleWellness.com
Join us at RodaleWellness.com/Join

© 2018 by Kerrilynn Pamer and Cindy DiPrima Morisse

Rodale books may be purchased for business or promotional use or for special sales. For information, please e-mail: BookMarketing@Rodale.com.

Printed in China

Rodale Inc. makes every effort to use acid-free ∞, recycled paper ♻.

Photographs by John von Pamer
Prop styling by Cindy DiPrima Morisse
Food styling by Victoria Granof

Book design by Rae Ann Spitzenberger

Library of Congress Cataloging-in-Publication Data is on file with the publisher.

ISBN 978-1-62336-972-9

Distributed to the trade by Macmillan

2 4 6 8 10 9 7 5 3   hardcover

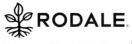

Follow us @RodaleBooks on 🐦 📘 📌 📷

We inspire health, healing, happiness and love in the world.
Starting with you.

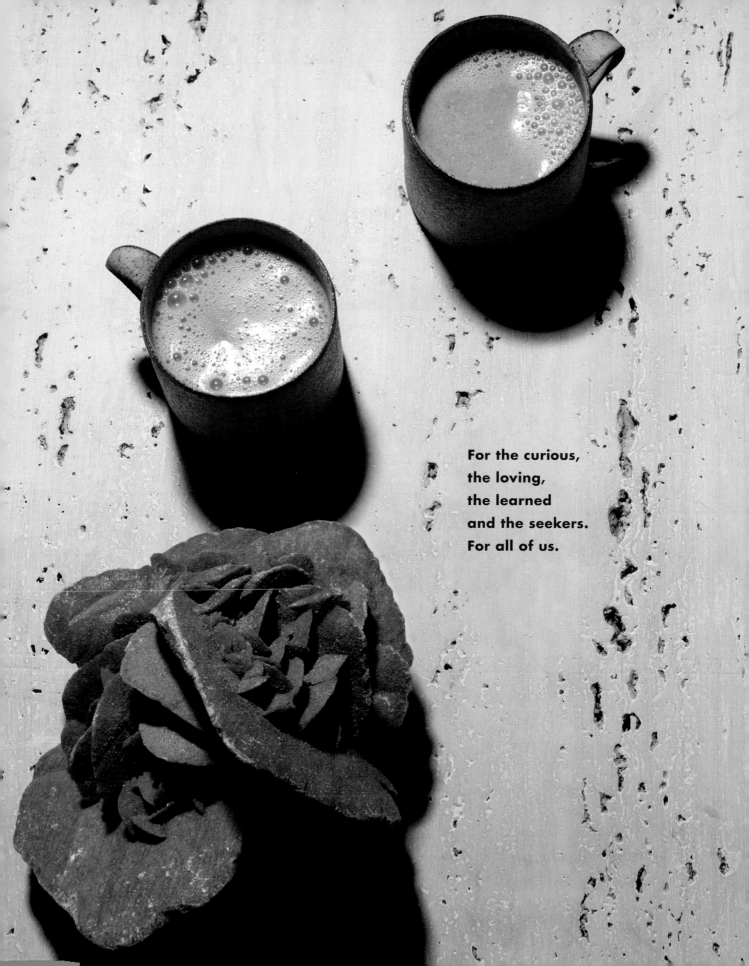

For the curious,
the loving,
the learned
and the seekers.
For all of us.

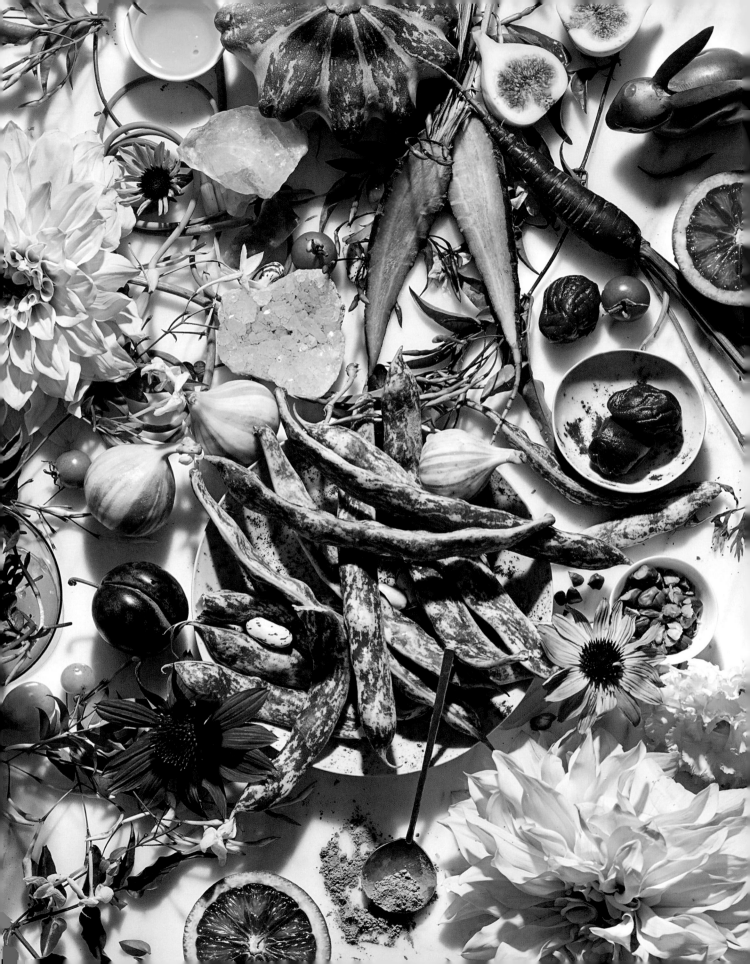

CONTENTS

INTRODUCTION

At CAP Beauty, we live by the motto that beauty is wellness. And, wellness is beauty. This applies to all aspects of our lives. From the books we read, to the foods we eat, to the homes we make, to the friendships we nurture, to the thoughts we play on repeat, beauty is all around. It stems from every choice we make. Embracing a life of conscious decisions, true self care and thoughtfulness connects you to beauty in a deep and meaningful way, one that transcends the physical. When we connect, we radiate. This is High Vibrational Beauty.

When we conceived of CAP Beauty, we envisioned a space to share this new beauty paradigm, a clubhouse where wellness rules and everyone's invited. Hailing from the worlds of style, design and magazines, we never considered ourselves beauty insiders.

And to this day, we focus as much on the lifestyle of natural beauty as we do on the products themselves. Don't get us wrong; we love an exquisite hydrosol, a powerful serum and a perfect lipstick. But, without ritual and true self care, a great product can only go so far. Step inside our world, where beauty meets beauty.

Our comprehensive approach engages all of our senses. You might be surprised to see so many recipes in a book about beauty. But for us, what we put in our bodies is as central to our beauty as what we put on our bodies. And, conversely, the products we use topically contribute to our inner health. This 360-degree approach means that we consider our food choices as much as we consider our skincare. We have a long-standing love for cooking, entertaining and sharing our love for nourishing foods, and we always welcome the chance to share a great recipe. Especially one that leaves us looking and feeling our best. So, when it comes to creating lasting beauty, we like to say, begin within.

And, since we're going beneath the surface, let's make one thing clear: We dive deep. It's in our nature. When we find something we love, we fall hard. We're self-proclaimed maximalists, and when it comes to healthy habits, we believe that more is more is more. Curiosity may have killed the cat but, for us, it's a way of life. There's so much to learn, so jump in. Lose the quick-fix mentality of a 3-day cleanse. This way of life is wildly fulfilling. And, as you take on your new healthy habits, you pave the way for more. You discover vitality and radiance on every level. Be kind to yourself, and remember this motto: progress not perfection.

Our beauty-meets-beauty approach stems largely from our backgrounds. We both came to beauty and wellness in our own time and way, as everyone's journey is unique.

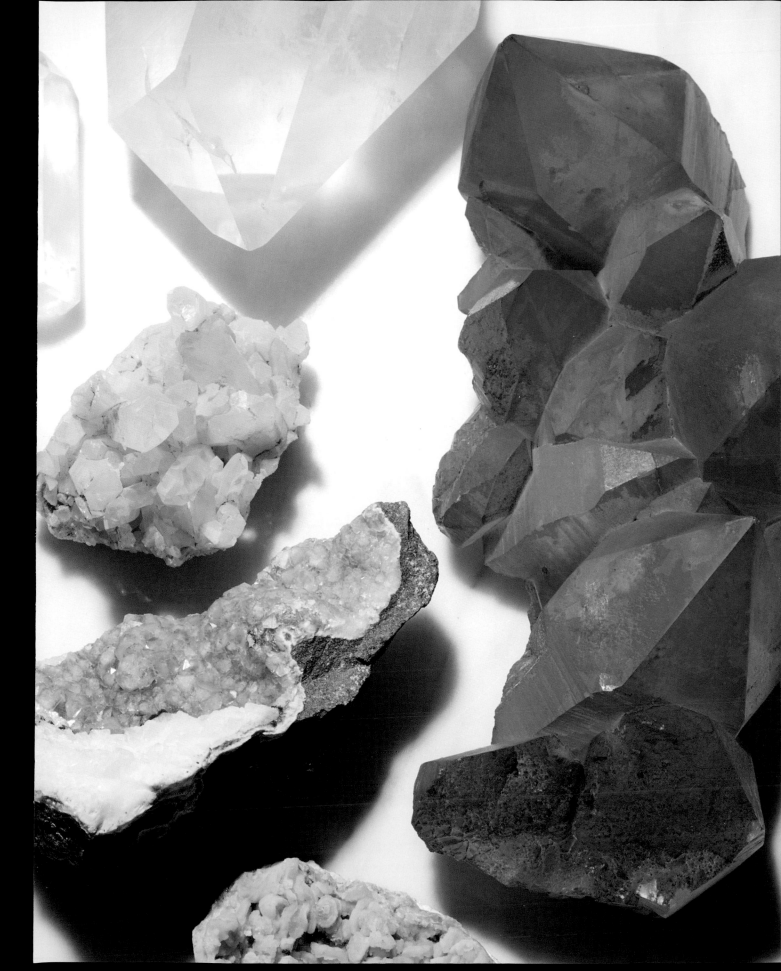

Cindy was largely influenced by her mom, Weezie, whose own interest in health and wellness stemmed from her upbringing on an apple farm. She emphasized the importance of natural foods and honoring the Earth, ecology and intricate cycles of life. Weezie followed the topics of the day, gleaning most of her knowledge from Jane Brody and the *New York Times*. Implementing these mainstream concepts into day-to-day life, she taught a young Cindy to recognize the importance of her choices. Cindy lost her mom to breast cancer when she was just 21. Weezie was 49. This precipitated an even deeper dive, and Cindy began her journey into a more esoteric and comprehensive interest in wellness. Of course, nothing happens overnight, and, for much of her young adulthood, this took the form of a late night out with friends followed by an early-morning yoga class, rich meals followed by a juice cleanse. A marriage and two kids later, her life is still an intricate work of balance. (Her husband, Laurent, is a wine dealer and an Ironman!) Armed with the knowledge from her childhood and her deeper dive into wellness, she works every day to share its power with her family and beyond.

Kerrilynn dove into wellness after being diagnosed with celiac disease almost a decade ago. She spent much of her childhood with unexplained stomach trouble and challenging skin issues that led her to doctors who suggested that she was simply unlucky or who prescribed antibiotics. When she finally discovered the root cause of it all, the skies parted. It all made sense, and she was thrilled to learn that feeling well was easily within reach. While many suggest that she's among the most unlucky for never being able to indulge in pizza, bagels and cake, Kerrilynn feels blessed and empowered. She's made it her life mission to share the knowledge that everyone has within them the power to feel good. Lifestyle choices and conscious decisions transformed her, and can transform us all. After giving up wheat, she slowly uncovered more ways to include wellness into her life. Cindy introduced her to Kris Carr, whose 21-day challenge led Kerrilynn to a life of plant-based eating. For her, this is the ticket to health and happiness. Herbs, fitness, Kundalini yoga, self-reflection, meditation and cleansing are all central to her well-being. She shares these practices at home with her husband, John, and her Puerto Rican rescue chihuahuas, but CAP Beauty is the portal for her to share them with the world.

WE OPENED THE DOORS TO A BEAUTY STORE, BUT UNKNOWINGLY LAUNCHED A LIFESTYLE BRAND.

We met each other while working at Martha Stewart Living, where we discovered our shared interests not only in wellness but also in style and gracious living. We are veterans of the design world where aesthetics rule. Just as beauty is more than skin-deep, how we live reflects our values. We opened the doors to a beauty store, but unknowingly launched a lifestyle brand. Because aesthetics are so deeply ingrained in us, it would be impossible to create a business that doesn't acknowledge all aspects of living. And, living beautifully.

When we set out to build our West Village store, we intended to create a space that was both aspirational and welcoming to all, a destination for the curious. We knew that natural beauty was no longer just for the hippie fringe. Yet, it still lived primarily in health food stores and yoga studios. Don't get us wrong, here. We love health food stores and yoga studios (more than you can imagine!), but our mission was to share these products with a larger audience, those not yet inducted into our "cult." We knew these sophisticated consumers were out there choosing natural and organic in almost all other areas of their lives, but since naturals lacked a modern and inspiring home, clean beauty was a holdout. Enter CAP Beauty.

By designing a store that was as visually stunning as it was pure in its mission, we appealed to this consumer, and we welcomed one and all. Every detail matters to us. As we built out our space, we embedded rose quartz under the floorboards to raise the vibration and encourage love. No one can see it, but everyone feels it. Even our contractor and his crew joined in, writing the Chinese characters for joy, love, health, wealth and happiness on the walls before painting. These invisible acts reverberate. They elevate and create a proper home for the deeply healing, nourishing and truly natural products that grace our shelves.

When we set the standards for what we would and wouldn't sell, we decided to keep it simple, and so we drew the line at 100 percent. That means that the products we stock use only natural ingredients and contain no synthetics at all. We've learned a lot since then, as this can certainly be a complex issue, and we work every day at maintaining this standard. It's central to our mission to be absolute and committed, creating a space of discovery, and one that is free from the confusion that so often surrounds the term natural.

Many people ask us for a list of the ingredients we don't carry, but frankly, we'd rather talk about the ones we do. Our products are teeming with active, transformative and truly magical plant ingredients, the building blocks of true beauty. We choose to focus on these.

And, we aren't missing anything. Often, the synthetics used in conventional beauty products are there to lengthen the shelf life or stabilize a product. Today's natural formulators find creative solutions to these very real issues. Since mold and harmful bacteria grow in water, many product developers simply eliminate the water, creating a product with a naturally longer shelf life. Powdered cleansers are a perfect example of this work-around. It's also why you'll notice more oils in the world of natural skincare. And, coincidentally (or we think not), oils relieve congested skin, naturally mimic our skin's sebum and are loaded with bioavailable nutrients. This is nature as it should be.

We encourage our customers to think of their products as they think of their food. Most of us would agree that a fresh peach is preferable to a canned peach, despite the obvious difference in shelf life. The fresh peach engages all of our senses and connects us to the Earth and to the season. Apply this thinking to your beauty routine, and watch your skin come alive. If a product is lingering in your medicine cabinet and not seeing the light of day, get rid of it. You shouldn't hold on for years on end (no matter how much it cost). Make space for the products you love, and use them. A long shelf life benefits business, not your skin. When you love your products and use them consistently, shelf life becomes irrelevant.

Another way we liken natural beauty to the world of food is by assessing our skin like we assess our hunger. Some days, you wake up hungry and need a hearty breakfast, whereas, other days, a green juice calls. Likewise, there are days when your skin will need more love than others. Some days, a deeper cleansing is in order, more hydration, a more active serum. Listen to your body; listen to your skin. Once you learn its language, you'll become fluent in what you need.

Clearly, we love food, making comparisons at every turn. So, it's natural we look to food to support our beauty from the inside out. What started as a tiny selection of products on our web site has grown into a thriving grocery corner that has a life of its own. By the time we opened our doors, we had a full shelving unit devoted to the herbs and superfoods we stock. And, our customers keep wanting more. We've been surprised (and yet not) by how popular these foods have become, and it thrills us when our customers make the connection between what they eat and how they look and feel. As we've said, it's impossible to separate beauty and wellness. And, what we eat is a cornerstone of health.

Education is vital to our mission. The world of natural beauty is advancing at lightning speed with so much information to distill. The products and practices we live by are new to many. And, to those already indoctrinated, there's always more to learn. So, we use our clubhouse as a classroom for free education. We enlist our own wellness heroes. Learning is vital to this lifestyle. Really, to any. Meditation, spirit animal quests, talks on adrenal health and tonic demonstrations are just some of the offerings in our curriculum. This component of CAP Beauty is so important to us that we hosted our first event just 2 days after we opened our doors. And, at every event, it thrills us to see the room fill up with busy New Yorkers (not known for their extra free time). We're inspired by the curious, and we count ourselves among them.

From the first days of visualizing CAP Beauty, we knew the importance of offering treatments. We think of our facials as another way to dive deep, and to learn and understand the nuances of skin and its health. At the time we opened, it was challenging to find a spa that offered truly natural facials. And, those that did relied on just one or two brands. We believe in the importance of diversity, of matching a client's skin to the perfect product. Because our estheticians can draw from so many product lines, they create a truly bespoke service for each and every one they see. Our clients learn to care for their skin on a deeper and more comprehensive level, and they learn the ever-important technique of facial massage, which is the backbone of our treatments. We teach our clients to understand that their skin is a living organ, one that is constantly shifting and reacting to the environment, both inside and out. It should be nurtured as such. Our CAP Beauty estheticians are like personal trainers for the skin, partners by your side to guide you to your most radiant self. Working out between training sessions is vital to improving fitness, and the self care you continue at home will yield the best results.

The CAP Beauty treatment had to embody our disruptive approach to conventional beauty, and so we enlisted a like-minded and brilliant expert in the field to write our protocol and educate our staff. Kristina Holey is unlike any skincare expert we've met. A true devotee to both science and self care, she views the skin as an ecosystem, one whose balance must be maintained through ritual, nutrition and topicals. She embodies our philosophy perfectly and, like us, dives deep. She

YOU'LL FEEL GREAT, AND, LIKE US, YOU'LL WANT TO SHOUT IT FROM THE ROOFTOPS.

brought her passion and intellect to CAP Beauty as well as her love for the extraordinary benefits of facial massage. You may be surprised to learn that simply massaging the skin can purify, detoxify, tone and oxygenate the skin to great effect. Expect vibrancy, hydration and the elusive glow. This is a pre-party facial. You don't need to schedule a night in. Go out and show it off.

The good news is, you can practice this technique at home and cultivate all of its benefits. And facial massage is just one of the rituals we offer in this book to deliver true health and radiance. When you adopt this High Vibrational Beauty lifestyle, your friends will take note. They might even just make you their guru. And, we say, share the love. You'll feel great, and, like us, you'll want to shout it from the rooftops.

Read on, and let beauty radiate from every aspect of your being.

THE HIGH VIBRATIONAL MANIFESTO

Natural beauty is a lifestyle, so much more than the products we buy and the ingredients they contain. It's the pursuit of raising our vibration on every level. These are the tenets we live by, the rules of the game for High Vibrational Living. These touchstones guide us, bringing truth and clarity to our daily choices. When our decisions align with our values, we access beauty on all levels.

EMBRACE THE POWER OF PLANTS

Mother Nature knows best. Let her bounty nourish you inside and out. Everything we need grows in her wild kingdom. Love your mother.

DIVE DEEP

Be curious, explore and go deep. Wellness is a marriage, not an afternoon fling. Commit to the power of commitment. Commit to your choices. Own them. Evolve with them. You're in this together.

CONSISTENCY CONQUERS

What we do every day counts more than what we do every once in awhile. When simple acts of self care become habit, we catalyze change. Focus less on the end goal and more on the acts that serve you daily. This is when true transformation happens.

CROWD OUT

Focus on adding in good habits and less on giving up the bad ones. When you commit to positive and healthy choices, there is simply less time and less desire for the patterns that don't serve you. Choose healthy abundance, not deprivation. And, welcome the shift.

MAKE SPACE

Clear the way. Making space creates clarity in mind and body. Get rid of what's weighing you down. Elevate to a higher state.

HONOR THE RHYTHMS OF NATURE

Live by the sun. Love by the moon. A deep connection to cycle informs your choices and rules self care. Be at one with the seasons. Succumb to what they ask. And, support yourself through daily, monthly and seasonal shifts.

BE PREPARED

Win the game before it even starts. With a little planning and prep, you set yourself up for victory each and every day. Claim the trophy.

STAND IN THE LIGHT

Embrace your life of change, and, as you raise your vibration, let it lift others. You won't need a soap box. The curious will find you. Stand in the light, and others will see.

MOVE AND SWEAT

Sweat it out to get it out. Sweating on the daily nurtures your body, mind and spirit. Few acts are as vital to our overall state of beauty. So, get moving. Free your mind and your toned a$$ will follow.

GET QUIET

Be still. Do it every day. Practice quiet, and experience a shift on every level.

FIND YOUR PURPOSE

When your mission is clear, life flows. Your North Star will light the way. Take the time to find yours. We all have one. Let it shine.

IN GRATITUDE

Give thanks for all you have. There's more to come, and then some. Love what you have, and the floodgates will open.

BE LOVE

It's all there is.

Welcome to our world of High Vibrational living. We put so much love and thought into the creation of this book and are so happy to see our beauty meets beauty vision come to life. We hope you love its pages, the images and the ideas. But, we also want you to use this book. And, use it hard. Don't be precious. It may be new and pristine right now, but we hope it doesn't stay that way. Our own most beloved books are dog-eared and tattered, stained from hours open on our kitchen counters. Dive in, get dirty and get High Vibe.

REASONS FOR THE SEASONS

Because we are so guided by the Earth's spin, we've organized the rituals in this book seasonally. Of course, there are many that you can and will practice daily, so don't be constrained by where they fall in the book. Certain rituals go hand-in-hand with particular seasons, but others go beautifully with all four. Discover with abandon, try them out and make your magic. Commit to the rituals that call your name. What works for your best friend may not be right for you. The important thing here is knowing yourself. Then, commit to your practice.

As we write this book, we live in New York City, where the seasons are pronounced. Where you live may be more temperate, with warmer winters and cooler summers, but there's always an energetic shift that the changing seasons bring. Connect to it, and embrace where you are. You're exactly where you should be.

The recipes in this book are developed to support you though the seasons. We tend to choose an abundance of raw, fresh fruits and vegetables in Summer months and gravitate toward grounding cooked foods as the temperatures drop. But, again, choose what your body craves.

IT'S ALL IN THE DETAILS . . . OR NOT

There's so much information in this book. Don't let it overwhelm you. Embrace this new way of life, and own it. But, don't be held hostage to every detail in the recipes and rituals. Interpret them in a way that works for you. Become the master of your kingdom. Improvise.

Our recipes contain many obscure and little known ingredients. As you embark further on this journey, they may become more familiar to you. You'll probably notice reference to them in the blogs you read and the podcasts you hear, as you get more into the High Vibrational lifestyle. And, you may grow increasingly curious. This is a good time to jump in.

But, we also know that time and budget may not allow for a full pantry makeover, so start where you can. If a shelf full of adaptogenic herbs is out of reach, make a pot of Kitcheree, a traditional mix of beans and rice that is used as a cleansing and detoxifying food in Ayurveda. When a recipe calls for something that you don't have on hand, try a substitution, or, in the case of adaptogens, like maca or reishi, just leave them out. You'll still be making a High Vibrational and nourishing meal. And, the simple act of cooking for yourself already puts you on the path.

As you become more fluent in these ingredients, you'll become comfortable swapping what is asked for with what you have on hand. This is how we cook. Don't let a missing ingredient stop you from creating a beautiful meal.

If you are ready to jump in and upgrade your pantry, start slowly. Use the Pantry Staples entry in the index to lead you. Bring home what speaks to you. You can also let a recipe inspire your purchases. Little by little, your pantry will transform. There's nothing better than a kitchen filled with life-giving and beautiful foods. Eat these in abundance, knowing that they align with your mission and elevate your body, mind and spirit. Healthy eating is joyful eating. Dig in.

FARMERS DO IT BETTER

Shop consciously. Whenever possible, we buy from our local farmer's market. Getting to know local growers allows for a deeper connection to the cycle of life. You'll discover new varieties and bring home fresher and more nutritious food, all while supporting their important work. And, they might just save you the best head of lettuce. Farming is hard, and we give eternal thanks to those who nourish us and the planet.

And, while we choose organic and encourage you to do the same, know that many growers may not have organic certification due to the often-prohibitive costs. But, they still may practice healthy and sustainable farming. If you're unsure, simply ask. Find out about their practices and their values, and decide if it's a match.

Buy the best ingredients your budget allows. Seek non-GMO, biodynamic and organic. We avoid gluten and dairy, but just because something is gluten free or vegan doesn't mean that it delivers health. So, be discerning. As we've said before, don't focus on what you're leaving out. Focus on what you're adding in. Look for whole food ingredients and eat foods that are as close to their natural state as possible. Our friend and nutritionist, Dana James, always says, "Eat only beautiful foods." It's that simple.

METHODS TO THE MINDFULNESS

THE KITCHEN TOOLS

We've tried to keep this accessible to all, with recipes anyone can make in a conventional home kitchen. But, if you want to go deep, there are upgrades and additions to the typical tools and equipment that most people have on hand. Some are affordable, and others are worth saving for. Here are the tools of our High Vibrational kitchens.

HIGH-SPEED BLENDER: Invest in the best, if you can. When you figure out your cost per use, even the most expensive blender will pay for itself, and then some. We love the American made Vitamix and its standard 7-year warranty. We're amazed to this day by how often we use this powerful machine. From our morning tonics to breakfast smoothies to raw pureed soups for lunch and dinner and even a batch of nut butter, a Vitamix in your kitchen is the easiest route to consuming an abundance of fruits and vegetables on the daily. Save a space for it on your counter. And, take it for a spin.

JUICER: Green juice is the holy water of High Vibrational living. And, when we embarked on this journey, a home juicer was essential. But, in the past decade or so, cold pressed juices have come into their own. They're mainstream now, and their availability has burgeoned. But, when time allows, we still love to press our own, customizing our very own blends and taking it straight from the source. There are countless varieties of juicers at a range of price points. Generally, the more expensive variety will yield a juice that oxidizes more slowly, meaning it will last longer in the fridge and hold onto its nutrients. Sometimes, the price can reflect ease of use, an important factor! Home juicing requires massive quantities of fresh fruits and vegetables, so make sure that you have the fridge space. And, if you take the dive, get creative. We love adding fresh herbs and biting tastes, like radish, to make juices that are truly our own.

AEROLATTE: This tiny throwback to the 1990s has a new life in our High Vibrational world of tonic drinks. Whip up your adaptogenic herbs, mushrooms and tocotrienols with a big spoonful of coconut butter for a new millennial latte.

DEHYDRATOR: Keep it alive! Dehydrating foods at at low temperatures keeps nutrients and vital minerals intact, making this an important addition to a raw food kitchen. Some use an oven, but a dehydrator allows for more control and multiple recipes to be prepared at once. Raw crackers, cookies and dried fruit are always on hand. Prepare for days-long "cooking" times and its lulling white noise. We've grown to love it.

NUT MILK BAG: This simple fabric bag is essential for straining the smoothest nut and seed milks. It's worth its modest price to avoid the mess of using a metal sieve, and the milk will come out its most refined. A tiny investment that you'll use all the time.

MANDOLINE: Another trick for helping us consume our lion's share of raw, living vegetables is to slice them finely and dress them well. Shaved vegetable salads are a staple in both of our homes. The mandoline makes it easy and fast. Countertop versions are great, but we also love the simple handheld style with a ceramic blade. It's also great for making vegetable chips.

BOX GRATER: Simple and old school, the box grater delivers. Grate carrots over your salads and zucchini over your soup. Up your dose of vegetables the easy way.

SPIRALIZER: Transform your vegetables. This remarkable tool spins vegetables into long spaghetti-like strands that can be lightly cooked or eaten raw. Your favorite sauce has a healthy new home.

FOOD PROCESSOR: Another investment piece, this is similar to a blender, and, in some cases, they're interchangeable. But, the nuanced differences are real, and they do offer slightly different results. The grater attachment makes grated salads fast and easy, and we definitely prefer a food processor for dips like hummus and our summertime favorite, Banana Nice Cream.

KNIVES: A beautiful knife is satisfying on all levels. When you eat more plants, chopping becomes a pastime. Make it one you enjoy. From France to Japan to Brooklyn, there's a knife for everything and everyone. Find one you love, and let it lead the way.

IMMERSION BLENDER: This low-investment piece purees cooked soups with minimal cleanup. Great for a small kitchen.

GLASS JARS AND STORAGE CONTAINERS: Decanting our High Vibrational staples (often purchased in the bulk aisle) serves more than just aesthetics. When ingredients live in stackable clear glass jars, we always know what's on hand. Take it a step further and shop with reusable muslin bags, so you can ditch the plastic. And, High Vibrational eating means that we often travel with a smoothie or soup packed to go, so we keep a stash of mason jars or recycled glass containers on hand. If you bake, choose wide-mouthed jars for your flours and other baking staples. This may seem unnecessary, like a purely aesthetic move, but it's a real game changer. You'll never wrestle with the mess of measuring again when you can easily get into the mouth of the jar.

MATCHA WHISK: This pretty Japanese tool elevates your matcha-making magic. You can easily swap it for a classic whisk or even a blender, but we love the ritual and feel of this beautiful tool.

THE KITCHEN PRACTICES

While classic cooking techniques apply to all diets, there are some tips that you'll lean on more when eating to raise your vibration. Here are some of our most used methods for maximizing nutrients and ease in the kitchen.

START EARLY: Get a head start. A little prep at breakfast time goes a long way toward getting dinner on the table. When time allows, we pull out our cutting boards and start chopping so that our evening meals are a seamless affair. Be your own sous chef, and prep what you can, so your post-work self has less to do. Even a few minutes in the morning can keep you from phoning in take-out at night.

MISE EN PLACE: The French know their way around the kitchen. You may have ditched the butter and cream, but keep this ingenious technique. Literally translating to "put in place," this method was made famous by TV chefs everywhere. Their little bowls of prepped ingredients are the key to cooking with confidence. When the prep is in place, you can enjoy the process, knowing nothing gets forgotten, and nothing gets burned. It may seem fussy, but it works. The joy of cooking starts here.

BATCH COOKING: There's something so satisfying about a Sunday spent preparing meals for the week. Big batches of soup, pots of beans and even veggies and fruits prepped for their final act. We love this approach, but often break it down throughout the week. Make a pot of quinoa on Monday, cook your beans on Tuesday, make a big carrot salad on Wednesday. This revolving door of nutritious building blocks lets us create dragon bowls and dinner salads at a moment's notice. Last minute entertaining becomes a reality when you have these staples on hand. Add fresh vegetables, oil-cured olives, sauerkraut and sprouted seeds, and dinner's done.

BE THE RAINBOW: Diversify and thrive. Eat as many colors as possible. If dinner is a big green salad, try gazpacho for lunch. Add color to your meals through the simplest of steps. Add grated carrots to your bowls, switch from white to purple onions, and choose red cabbage over white. Anywhere you can, add color. You'll be adding vital nutrients and fiber in the process. And, your plate will be a beautiful rainbow.

SOAKING: Soaking beans can greatly reduce their cooking time, and soaking nuts before making milks can be easier on the blender, but soaking can also make these foods more digestible and their nutrients more bioavailable. Expect to always have a bowl of something soaking on the counter, little reminders that a healthy meal is in process. These are nourishing traditions for the plant-based world. When soaking beans, we add a piece of Kombu (a type of sea kelp) to add minerals and further help with digestion. So, plan ahead, and soak it in.

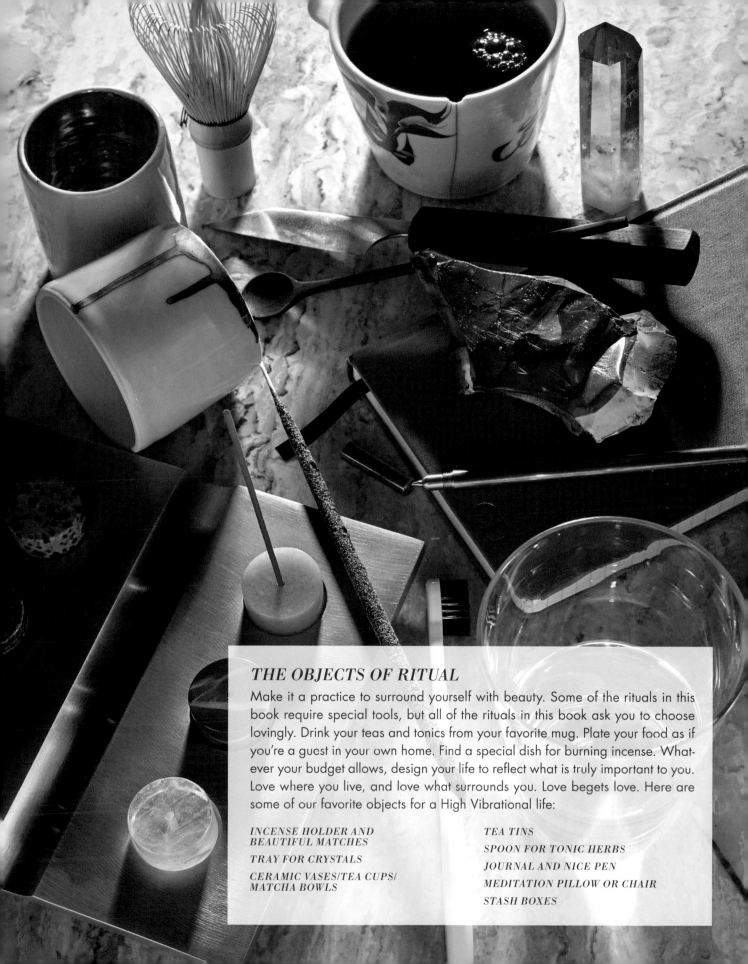

THE OBJECTS OF RITUAL

Make it a practice to surround yourself with beauty. Some of the rituals in this book require special tools, but all of the rituals in this book ask you to choose lovingly. Drink your teas and tonics from your favorite mug. Plate your food as if you're a guest in your own home. Find a special dish for burning incense. Whatever your budget allows, design your life to reflect what is truly important to you. Love where you live, and love what surrounds you. Love begets love. Here are some of our favorite objects for a High Vibrational life:

INCENSE HOLDER AND
BEAUTIFUL MATCHES

TRAY FOR CRYSTALS

CERAMIC VASES/TEA CUPS/
MATCHA BOWLS

TEA TINS

SPOON FOR TONIC HERBS

JOURNAL AND NICE PEN

MEDITATION PILLOW OR CHAIR

STASH BOXES

SPRING

AN INTRO TO SPRING: THE REAWAKENING

For us, spring is possibility. After the chill and quietude of winter, we embrace its new growth. A return to sun-kissed days, lighter foods and more time outdoors makes spring a season to celebrate. We are reborn, rekindling our deep love affair with Mother Earth. We plant in her soils, roll in her grasses and dance in her rains. We know in our hearts that, for the next half-year, our bodies will be warm, and our spirits will be light. Longer days and sultry nights, we welcome you.

The recipes and rituals shared here are designed to prepare your body, mind and spirit for a reawakening. The season of rebirth lies ahead. Embrace it.

BEAUTY

THE SPRING SKIN PROGRAM

PERFORM: Once or twice daily

WHAT YOU'LL NEED: Cleanser, toner and oil or moisturizer

DURATION: 5 to 10 minutes

Put your best face forward, and shine bright like a diamond. Incorporating a deep and thorough cleansing ritual into your bedtime routine will encourage your most beautiful skin ever. While we sleep, our skin detoxes, moving toward perfect balance, so everything we can do to support our skin before bed is beneficial. A thorough cleanse, a deep massage and a sealing of moisture leaves you glowing and radiant. Evenings are the focus of our skincare regimens. By committing to a more thorough cleansing routine at night, you allow your body's natural rhythms to support your most radiant and nourished skin. A deep cleanse and massage encourages overnight cellular regeneration and healing, making a simpler, more streamlined routine in the morning. Many mornings, you can even skip the cleanse and just do a quick wake up with cold water, a spritz of hydrosol and a moisturizer or serum. We encourage you to cleanse the moment you get home. As busy women, we know all too well that the evening can be taken up with other obligations, and sleep can set in all too fast. By taking care of your skin early on, your most active products have a longer time to work, and you have more time to relax. Another one of our favorite self care activities. And, best of all, washing your face won't fall by the wayside. Sweet dreams, natural beauties.

After the long chill of winter many of us are left dry and sensitive. Spring's rainy climate is a welcome shift. Your routine these months incorporates revitalizing nutrient-dense products that hydrate with a lighter hand. Those with less sensitive skin will also look to exfoliate, to remove the layers of winter. Through the foods we eat and the products we choose, we also start to prepare our skin for more time spent outside, laying the groundwork for healthy time in the sun.

HOW TO DO IT: Start with a small amount of cleanser in your hand, and apply it to the skin on your face. Work into your neck and face for 2 to 4 minutes, using small and gentle circular motions moving upward from the neck to the forehead, spending extra time on the center of your face. Do your best to not rush through the massage. Take care, but massage your face like you mean it. Facial massage increases blood flow, oxygenates muscle tissues and assists in the flow of the lymphatic system, revealing a healthy and youthful glow. Then, add some water to your fingertips and work it into your skin, removing your cleanser. Continue this part for 2 to 3 minutes, incorporating enough water to remove all of the cleanser. Do not use hot water. Warmish is best. Make sure that all the cleanser is removed, and softly blot your face with a soft, clean towel.

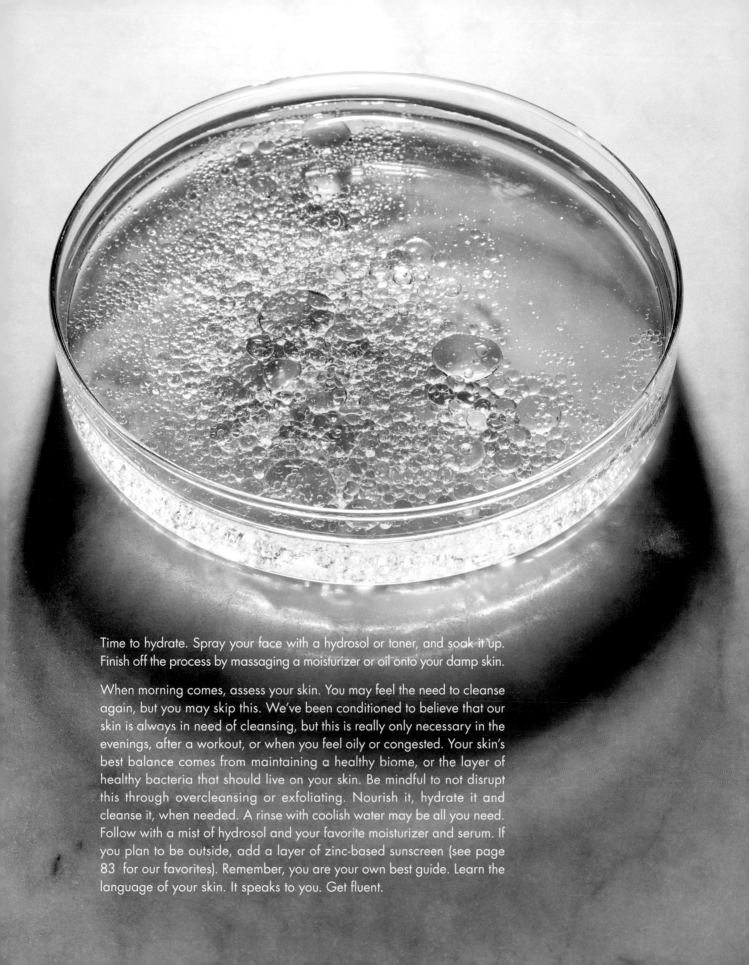

Time to hydrate. Spray your face with a hydrosol or toner, and soak it up. Finish off the process by massaging a moisturizer or oil onto your damp skin.

When morning comes, assess your skin. You may feel the need to cleanse again, but you may skip this. We've been conditioned to believe that our skin is always in need of cleansing, but this is really only necessary in the evenings, after a workout, or when you feel oily or congested. Your skin's best balance comes from maintaining a healthy biome, or the layer of healthy bacteria that should live on your skin. Be mindful to not disrupt this through overcleansing or exfoliating. Nourish it, hydrate it and cleanse it, when needed. A rinse with coolish water may be all you need. Follow with a mist of hydrosol and your favorite moisturizer and serum. If you plan to be outside, add a layer of zinc-based sunscreen (see page 83 for our favorites). Remember, you are your own best guide. Learn the language of your skin. It speaks to you. Get fluent.

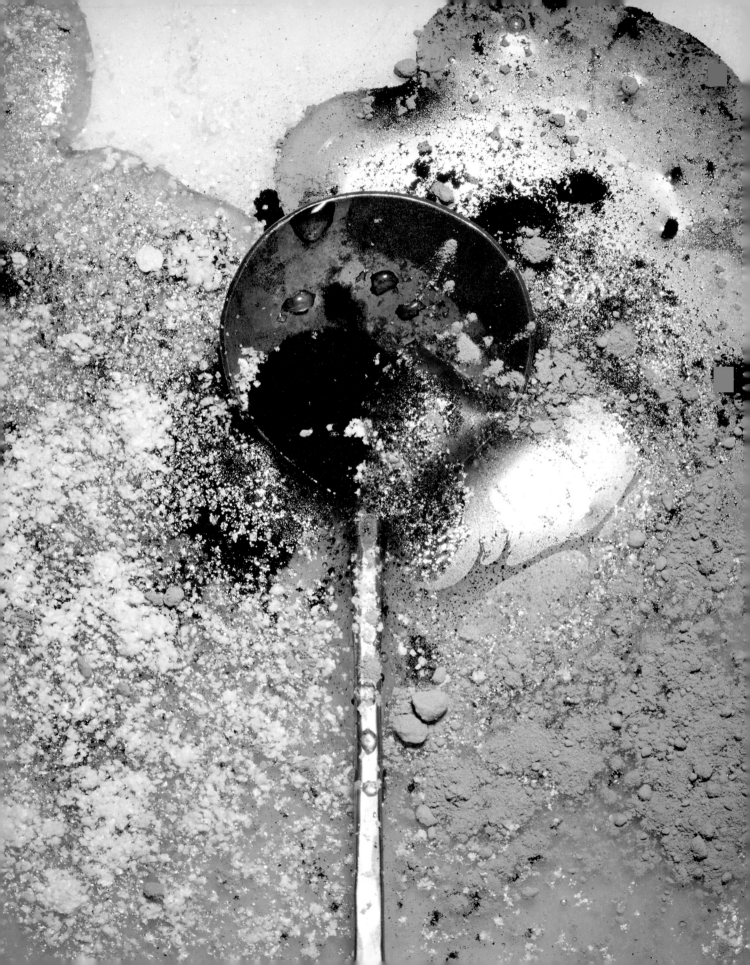

A REPLENISHING MASK FOR BRIGHTER DAYS

Our love for a good mask runs deep. We love the range that we sell at CAP Beauty, with something for every season and every skin type. But, we also love to get in the kitchen and formulate our own, using staples from our superfood pantry, confirming our belief that the best skincare mimics a healthy diet, with nutrients at the forefront and only pure and life-giving ingredients. As you dive deeper into this book, you'll learn to understand your skin and care for it lovingly and intuitively. Mixing these masks will become second nature. Channel your inner chef, and your skin will thank you.

This mask contains high levels of antioxidants and vitamins D and E, is anti-inflammatory, purifying, calming and has gently exfoliating properties. It's perfect for the season, as it helps to shed winter layers while nourishing and feeding your skin. Of course, it's clean enough to eat. (And, most likely, delicious!)

HOW TO DO IT: Whisk or stir ½ teaspoon matcha into 1 tablespoon water and set aside. Add to a small ceramic bowl ½ tablespoon tocotrienols, 1 tablespoon honey and 1 teaspoon chlorella and mix well with the brush. Slowly and deliberately pour the brewed matcha, as needed, until it reaches a pastelike consistency. Be careful not to create too thin a consistency. If needed, add more tocotrienols and honey.

Apply to your clean face with the brush. Allow to sit for 20 minutes. We like to take a bath or meditate while we're masking. It may be drippy, so lying down is smart. Enjoy a timeout.

Remove with warm or cool water, scrubbing gently to promote a light exfoliation. Your skin will feel dewy, cleansed and revived.

PERFORM:
Once a week,
two times is great

WHAT YOU'LL NEED:
Matcha, water, tocotrienols, manuka honey, chlorella, a small ceramic bowl and brush

DURATION:
20 to 30 minutes

SPRING PRODUCT RECOMMENDATIONS

CLEANSER: Mūn Akwi Purifying Cleanser, Marie Veronique Gentle Gel Cleanser, African Botanics Baobab Clay Oxygenating Cleanser

HYDROSOL: Hannes Dottir Mineral Mist, Marie Veronique Pre + Probiotic Daily Mist, Living Libations Rose Glow Complexion Mist

MOISTURIZER: Tata Harper Repairative Moisturizer, May Lindstrom The Blue Cocoon, Leahlani Bless Beauty Balm

SERUM: Leahlani Champagne Serum, In Fiore Complexe de Fleur, One Love Organics Morning Glory Caffeinated Firming Serum

DRY BRUSHING

PERFORM:
Once daily, two
times is great

WHAT YOU'LL NEED:
Dry brush

DURATION:
5–10 minutes

Strip down and brush up. Dry brushing detoxifies, beautifies and energizes. This practice assists the lymphatic system and stimulates circulation while brilliantly exfoliating the body from head to toe. The lymphatic system is a vital component of immune function and detoxification that rids the body of waste and toxins. "Lymph" is the Latin word for water. And, water is life.

HOW TO DO IT: Get in your bathtub or next to your tub. Using your clean, dry brush, begin at your ankles and brush the skin in long upward strokes. It is important to always move the brush in the direction of your heart. Start at the inside of the legs and move to the side, the back and then the insides again. Do not scrub the body with your brush, just move in one consistent direction toward your center. Spend some extra time on the back of the legs and backside. Move to the lower back and belly, and continue your long upward strokes. Next, hold an arm out and begin strokes at the wrist. Start at the inside of each arm and move toward the top, the back and the inside again, still moving up toward your heart. Now, reach behind you and dry brush the upper back and shoulders using outward strokes. Finally, do the same to the top of your chest (do not brush the delicate skin of your breasts), brushing out toward the armpits.

NOTES: We recommend cleaning your dry brush at least once a week, but make sure it's fully dry before your brushing ritual the next day. Clean with hot water and hang to dry in a nonhumid place. We like a sunny window.

THE SPRING BATH

PERFORM:
Once a week
is ideal

WHAT YOU'LL NEED:
Your favorite
bath salts

DURATION:
10–20 minutes

Bathe yourself in holy water and be born again. A true act of self-love, bathing nourishes the body, mind and spirit. Salt baths (Epsom and Dead Sea salts are among our favorites) infuse the body with magnesium and other vital minerals, soothing sore muscles, encouraging better sleep and fighting inflammation.

HOW TO DO IT: Burn your Palo Santo or favorite incense and prepare for your soak. Fill the tub with hot water, and visualize it healing your body. Add the salts to the bath (we like a cup to two cups of Epsom salt). Swirl the salt around the tub, step in and slowly lower yourself into the water. Lie back and relax for 10 to 20 minutes, while listening to a guided meditation. When you feel thoroughly relaxed, exit the bath and wrap yourself up in a thick towel. Then, go rest and take in the transformative and healing properties of the salt.

NOTES: Buy several large cartons of Epsom salt at your local drugstore. They're inexpensive and easy to find.

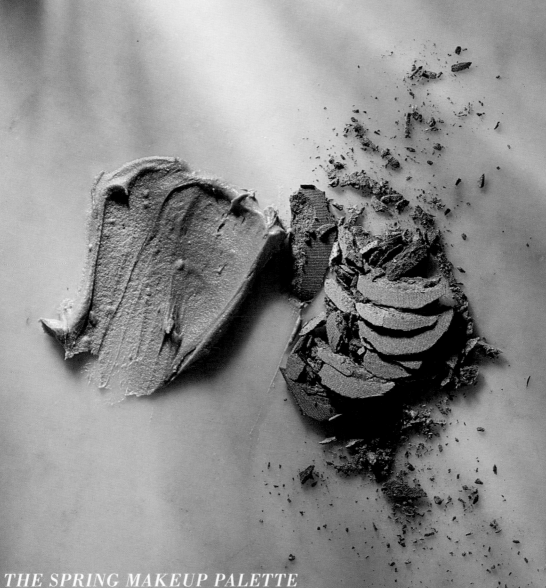

THE SPRING MAKEUP PALETTE
Lighten up and reveal your softer side. Inspired by new growth, new beginnings and the hopeful light of spring, we gravitate toward yellows, greens and blush tones, the very colors handed to us by Mother Nature. Our skin reunites with the sun, and we welcome the warm glow that follows. Highlight and embrace these tones, and let your colors reflect this season of opportunity.

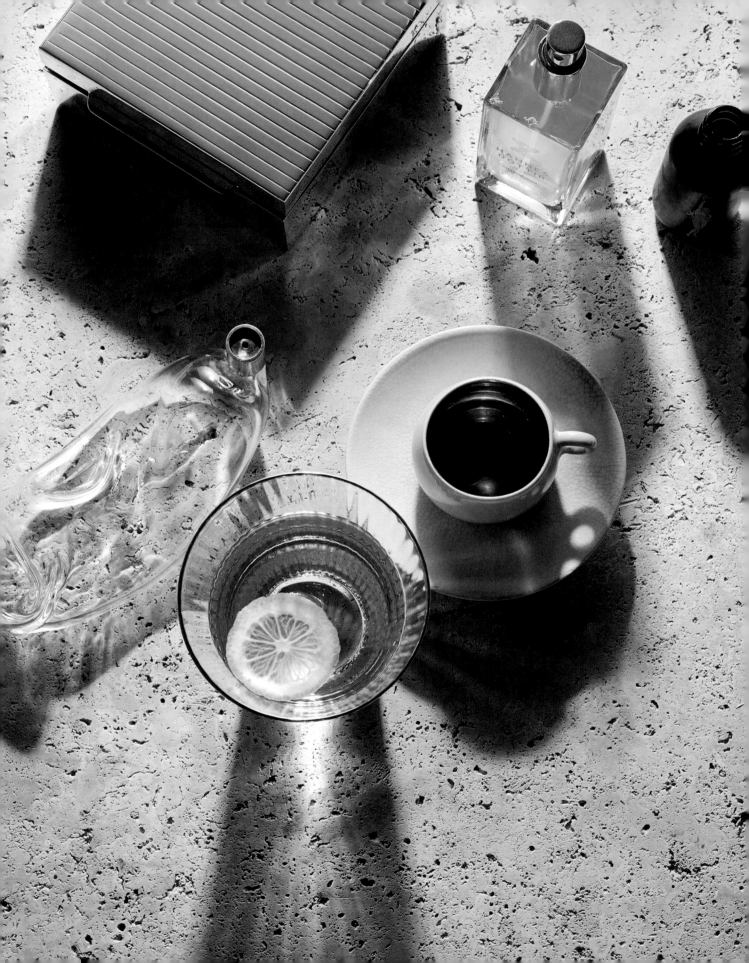

BODY

CINDY'S MORNING RITUAL MAGIC

Harness the magic of the morning. By beginning our days with a steady routine of rituals and rites, we set our intentions and ensure that each day embraces the gifts of self care. And, while consistency is key, our routines vary from season to season. Our springtime morning rituals help us ease back into the warmer months. We welcome transformation, encouraging our bodies to draw nourishment from the gifts of light.

Here's how Cindy begins her day:

"I wake up minutes before the alarm clock rings at 6:00 a.m. Waking at this hour allows me to enjoy a few precious moments before my husband and kids wake up. Before I even get out of bed, I spend a moment or two reminding myself what's on the agenda for the day, counting my blessings and asking the universe for what I want and need. Then, I practice 22 minutes of transcendental meditation. Next, I head to the kitchen, where I down a big glass of room temperature filtered water with lemon and a couple of probiotics. I turn on the kettle, and make lunch for the kids. When the lunches are packed, I make a carafe of organic coffee in the Chemex that my husband, Laurent, and I share. I love a small cup of dark roast coffee, and always take it black. Some mornings, I'll fit in a run or interval style sprints. Other mornings, I relax and catch up with Laurent. Quinton shots (straight shots of purified ocean water), packs of LivOn vitamin C and a simple skincare routine come next. I head to the office around 9:00 and usually stop on the way to pick up a green juice that I'll have as breakfast.

MASSAGE

The power of touch is in your hands. And, everything you touch turns to gold. Rooted in Abhyanga, the ayurvedic practice of self-massage, this ritual encourages a deep love for yourself, your body and your beautiful skin. Massage stimulates circulation and combats stress by increasing endorphin levels and lowering cortisol. Oxygenate your muscles, boost lymphatic drainage and feel your best.

HOW TO DO IT: Warm the oil by placing the bottle in a bowl or sink filled with hot water. In the meantime, rinse your bathtub with hot water to warm it up. When the oil feels good to the touch, get undressed and stand in the bathtub or a warm room. Start at your feet and begin massaging the oil into your skin. Work your way up the body with long, firm strokes, ending at the neck. Use circular motions on your joints (ankles, knees, hips, shoulders, elbows). Take time with the process, the results are in the journey. Let the oil penetrate the skin for at least 20 minutes. Enjoy your downtime. Follow with a bath or shower.

PERFORM:
Once daily, in the evenings or when you aren't rushing out the door

WHAT YOU'LL NEED:
Massage oil

DURATION:
10–30 minutes

WARMING IT UP

PERFORM: Daily

WHAT YOU'LL NEED:
Motivation, discipline
and your favorite
workout gear

DURATION:
20 minutes to
2 hours daily
for 5 or 6 days

Transformation starts here. The power of movement never fails to amaze us. By moving your body, you encourage the fastest and most profound shift in your physical and mental state. Nearly every aspect of well-being is enhanced through regular exercise. As the temperature rises, and the days get longer, we return to daily movement. We're all about feeling good in our bodies at any time of year, and by all means, we encourage regular movement through all seasons, but the sleepier tones of winter can sometimes derail us. Spring is an ideal season to recommit.

GETTING STARTED: If you have a regular exercise habit, just get back to it. If you're starting from scratch, here are some ideas to ease you into this way of life.

CONSISTENCY FIRST: We wholeheartedly believe in the power of consistency in exercise and in any wellness practice. Running a half-marathon once a year will not benefit you on the daily. A practice that gets you moving each day will change you. This has been a profound revelation for both of us, and truly has changed our approach to exercise and every aspect of High Vibrational living. It's what you do each day that counts. We also live by the well-known motto that perfection is the enemy of done. So, if you miss a day, don't sweat it. Just get back in the game tomorrow. An intentional rest day can also do wonders for the body, and it's part of practicing consistency.

COMMITTED MOVEMENT: When you're working out, give it what you have. Sweat it out, and learn to push yourself. This doesn't mean jumping in the deep end if you don't know how to swim. But, whatever your level, find your edge. You'll know it when you get there. And, if you have a hard time pushing yourself, find a partner or go to a class. Accountability is a mighty force. On the flip side, when you're resting, take it as seriously as when you're working out. Give your body the space to recover. Listen, it will tell you.

DIVERSIFY: Just like with the foods we eat, it's important to mix it up. By incorporating different forms of movement, you engage your mental and physical self, challenge different muscle groups and increase your overall fitness. We love to alternate between yoga, running, HIIT, dance class, Pilates, a vigorous walk and playing sports (hello, tennis!). There's a time and place for all, and mixing it up is a lot more fun. Leave your comfort zone. Try something new, and welcome the transformation.

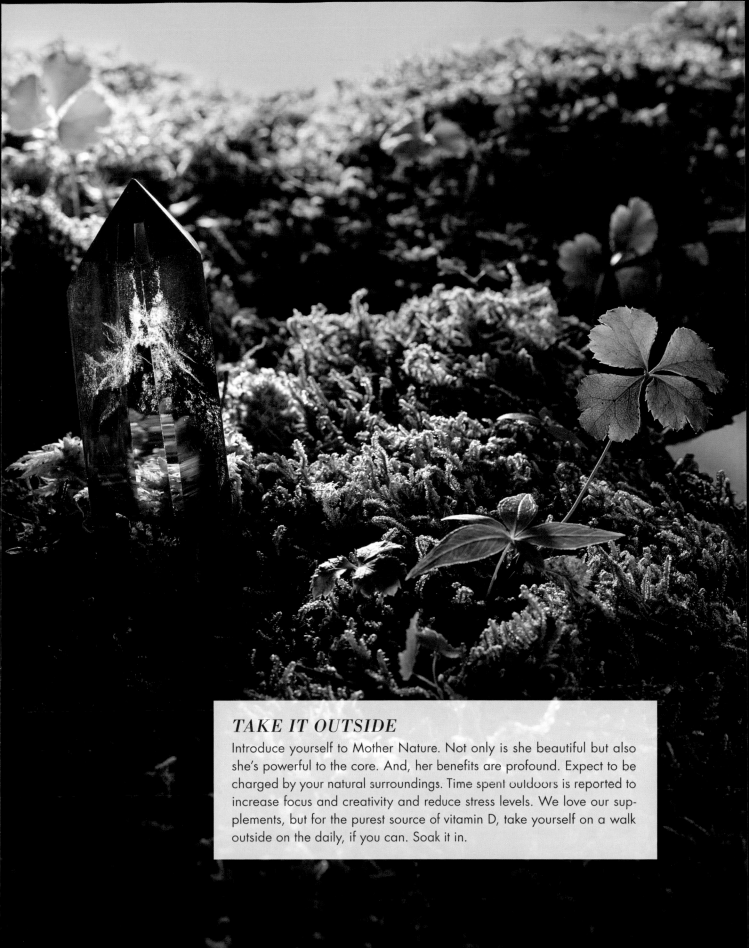

TAKE IT OUTSIDE

Introduce yourself to Mother Nature. Not only is she beautiful but also she's powerful to the core. And, her benefits are profound. Expect to be charged by your natural surroundings. Time spent outdoors is reported to increase focus and creativity and reduce stress levels. We love our supplements, but for the purest source of vitamin D, take yourself on a walk outside on the daily, if you can. Soak it in.

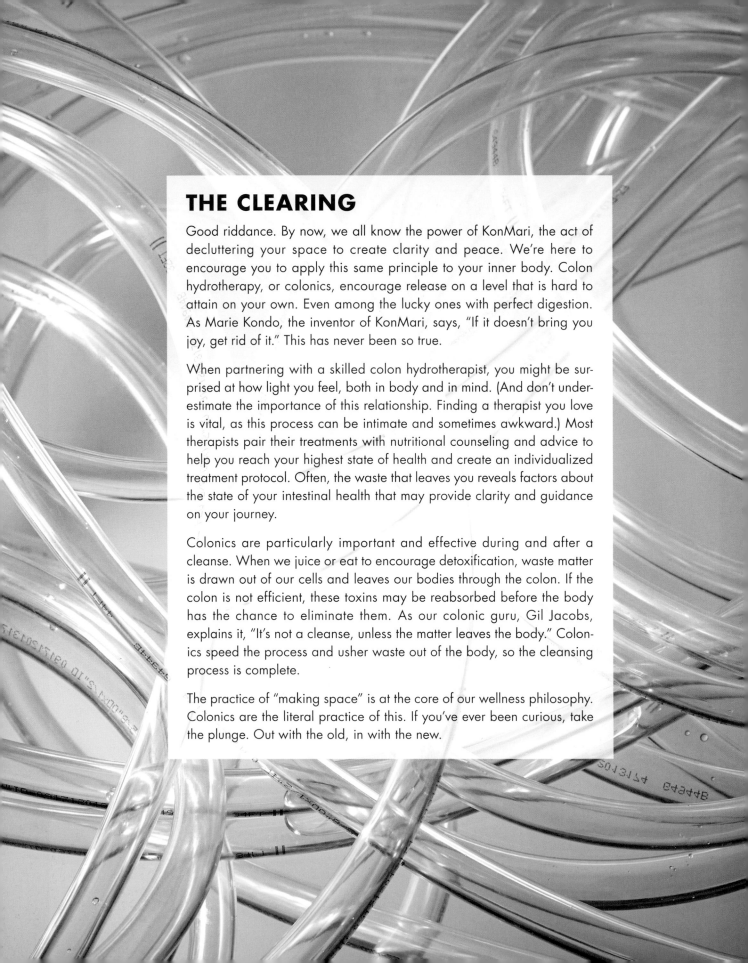

THE CLEARING

Good riddance. By now, we all know the power of KonMari, the act of decluttering your space to create clarity and peace. We're here to encourage you to apply this same principle to your inner body. Colon hydrotherapy, or colonics, encourage release on a level that is hard to attain on your own. Even among the lucky ones with perfect digestion. As Marie Kondo, the inventor of KonMari, says, "If it doesn't bring you joy, get rid of it." This has never been so true.

When partnering with a skilled colon hydrotherapist, you might be surprised at how light you feel, both in body and in mind. (And don't underestimate the importance of this relationship. Finding a therapist you love is vital, as this process can be intimate and sometimes awkward.) Most therapists pair their treatments with nutritional counseling and advice to help you reach your highest state of health and create an individualized treatment protocol. Often, the waste that leaves you reveals factors about the state of your intestinal health that may provide clarity and guidance on your journey.

Colonics are particularly important and effective during and after a cleanse. When we juice or eat to encourage detoxification, waste matter is drawn out of our cells and leaves our bodies through the colon. If the colon is not efficient, these toxins may be reabsorbed before the body has the chance to eliminate them. As our colonic guru, Gil Jacobs, explains it, "It's not a cleanse, unless the matter leaves the body." Colonics speed the process and usher waste out of the body, so the cleansing process is complete.

The practice of "making space" is at the core of our wellness philosophy. Colonics are the literal practice of this. If you've ever been curious, take the plunge. Out with the old, in with the new.

CLEANSING

We've seen the cleanse go from fringe to mainstream, and, while many embrace it for its promise of weight loss and glowing skin, we also love a cleanse for its clearing of the psyche and the resetting of habits. Through the disciplined practice of drinking only juices (or soups and smoothies), we change our relationship to hunger and the foods we eat. And, by giving our bodies a rest from the taxing practice of digestion, we encourage a deeper state of relaxation in the body. This practice has transformed the way that Cindy and Kerrilynn approach health and wellness. Simple, yet not easy, but so effective for a total reset of body and mind. Your detox starts here.

The warmer seasons lend themselves to an easier cleanse. Abundant produce and sunlight make spring and summer ideal for juicing and consuming more raw foods.

There are all different theories about how and when to cleanse. Some prefer only juices, others mix in blended drinks and even solid food (usually raw and vegan). Some go for weeks, and even months. Others like to cleanse a day or two every week. Depending on where you are in your journey, it's important not to dive in too deep too fast. Use relativity as your guiding light. The concept is not to radically transform yourself with a week of juicing. The idea, instead, is to begin a practice of periodic cleansing. Let the cumulative benefits build and move steadily toward a state of true health.

One of our favorite benefits of cleansing is the release from a nearly constant focus on food. As two food-lovers, we spend a lot of time discussing and planning our meals. This is, in fact, one of our great joys, but it's also great to take a break. When cleansing, all variables are off the table. Breakfast, lunch and dinner are designed, and we can move on to other topics. The first day can be a challenge, even the second, but, with time, your body becomes accustomed to the practice, and even craves it.

A note on deprivation. This is all a state of mind. Shift your mindset to see the power of what you're doing for your body. Flooding yourself with vital, life-giving nutrients is an awesome form of self-love. You'll feel and see the benefits from brighter skin and eyes to a flatter tummy and a deep sense of pride. You'll feel rested and alive. You got this.

PERFORM:
Weekly, monthly, or seasonally

WHAT YOU'LL NEED:
Determination

DURATION:
1 day to 1 week

RAISING KUNDALINI ENERGY: SAT KRIYA

PERFORM:
Once daily

WHAT YOU'LL NEED:
A timer, a quiet room
and an open mind

DURATION:
3 minutes, to start

Sat Kriya is the primary practice to raise Kundalini energy. What does that mean? Kundalini energy lives in all of us, but is dormant in most. Simple practices called Kriyas are designed to awaken this powerful energy through breathwork, mantras and repetitive movement. More than likely, you won't hear about the benefits of Kundalini from your doctor, trainer or science teacher, but we know from practice that it is powerful beyond measure. And, we're not the only ones on board. Kundalini yoga is gaining momentum for its ability to create deep transformation and clear blockages. It works, and it works quickly. Open your mind, and welcome the change.

Kundalini is a perfect addition to your beauty routine, as it moves energy, dissipates stagnancy and gives a clear, enlightened gaze and a radiance from within.

Sat Kriya can be practiced for just 3 minutes, but experienced yogis build up to longer sessions of 7, 11, 22 or 31 minutes. These specific increments are considered to be sacred numbers shared by Yogi Bhajan, who brought Kundalini to the West in the 1970s. And, remember, even a short session yields great change.

HOW TO DO IT: Sit in Rock Pose, simply kneeling on your feet. If this is uncomfortable, sit in a simple cross-legged position. Stretch your arms above your head with no bend in your elbows. Your upper arms should be next to your ears. Interlace your fingers and extend your index fingers pointing toward the sky. Your thumbs should be crossed with your left thumb on top for women and your right thumb on top for men. Close your eyes and gaze toward your third eye or slightly above your eyebrows.

When you're ready to begin, set your timer for 3 minutes. Start to chant "Sat Nam" (pronounced Sut Naam) in sync with your breath. As you say "Sat," squeeze your navel toward your spine, working carefully not to let the rest of your body move with it (isolate your abdomen). Release your belly while chanting "Nam." Repeat at a moderate pace until your time is up.

To finish, inhale deeply and with your breath held in, apply root lock. Known to some as Mula Banda, this is a contraction of the sex organs and a lift and engagement of the pelvic floor. Think Kegel exercises, and visualize the Kundalini energy moving up your spine and out through your fingertips. Hold for roughly 10 seconds and exhale. Do this closing breath three times. If time allows, lie down in Corpse Pose for an additional 3 minutes. Feel the change in your energy.

HARNESSING SOURCE ENERGY

Harmonize with your higher power. We all have one. At CAP Beauty, we talk a lot about vibrational energy, and getting high with it. Surfer talk aside, there is reason behind this pursuit. Everything on this great Earth contains energy, and vibrates at some frequency. Roses, for example, are one of the highest vibrational flowers in the plant kingdom. And, so, it's no wonder that they are one of the most widely used ingredients in natural beauty. They are also an icon for love, and one of the most beloved and symbolic flowers in the world. When we raise our vibration, we find ourselves attracting other High Vibrational people and things. Like attracts like, and this couldn't be more true than with the vibrational pull of other beings.

You may call it God, the universe, or simply your higher power, but Source is simply the unlimited flow of divine energy. It is a wellspring of possibility, and it is infinite. When we align our own energy with Source, we enter a state of flow and grace. We tap into this resource when our intentions are clear and our motivations are pure. For us, knowing and witnessing the power of Source has been profound and humbling. When we conceived of CAP Beauty, we weren't aware that so many of our successes would spring from this higher place. One of the first projects we did as a company was to draft a manifesto, a sort of North Star that would spell out our mission. This simple document guides us, governs our partnership and brings a sense of knowing into every decision we face. Cindy used to say that it didn't feel like we were building CAP Beauty, but simply shepherding it into the world. At other times, when the going is good, we've joked that "This is so easy!" Of course, it's not, but it is filled with ease. Because Source is on our side.

Tapping into this higher power is a fundamental and prominent theme in everything we do. To access Source energy, start with a heavy dose of faith. This might feel out there. But, a great place to start is to think of times in your life that you've received exactly what you needed, whether you knew it at the time or not. Hindsight is 20/20, especially when you're counting your blessings.

Another important way to connect to Source is to make sure that your "ask" aligns with the higher good. You don't need to start a not-for-profit or solve world hunger, but you should believe that what you're creating contributes in a positive way. And, remember that simply living your purpose is a way to enhance the world and is a direct line to the power of Source.

The connection to Source should be constantly nourished. Choose activities and friends that enrich you. Raise your vibration through healthy eating, moving your body, quieting your mind and getting outside into nature. Practice gratitude, and remind yourself on the daily that the universe has your back. This ability to tap in and to believe in Source energy is like a muscle. The more you use it, the stronger it grows.

CRYSTALS FOR BALANCE

These are the stones we keep on hand to balance energies, physically and spiritually. Some will also help to release old patterns and encourage the new growth of spring.

TURQUOISE: This native beauty acts as a buffer and a guide.

CHRYSOCOLLA: This green stone encourages true expression.

CHRYSOPRASE: The stone of Libra, the zodiac master of balance, brings fortune and fertility.

SODALITE: This deep-blue stone rules communication and logic.

EMERALD: Brilliant and green, emeralds are the stone of love and domestic bliss.

JADE: Receive luck and blessings from this dream stone.

MOONSTONE: This powerful mistress enhances the feminine divine.

MALACHITE: This master of business encourages success and lends its hand in balancing relationships.

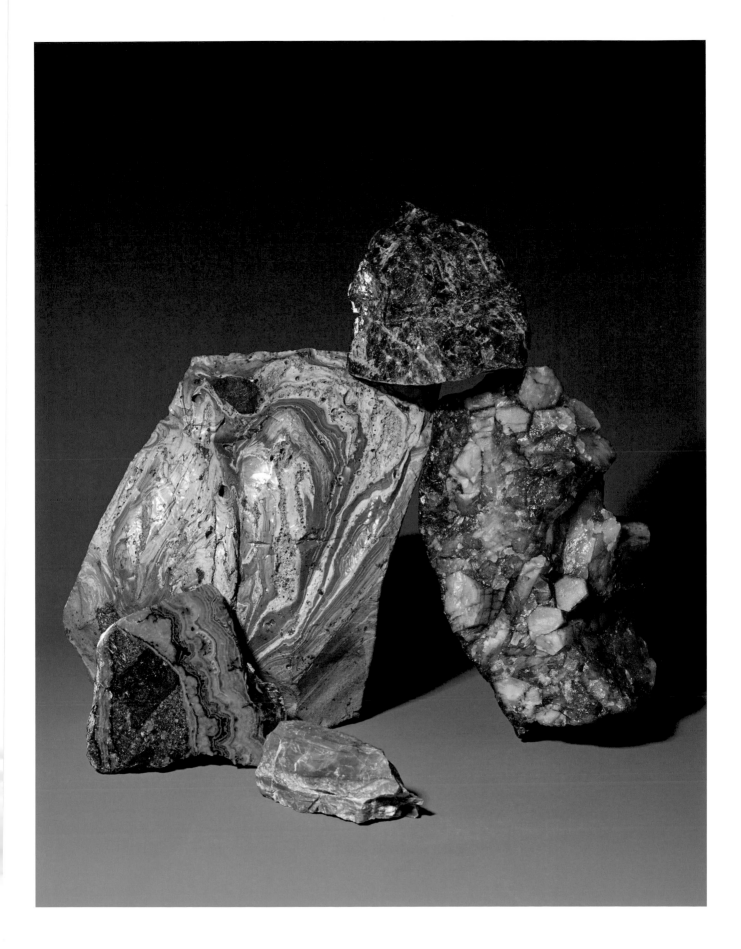

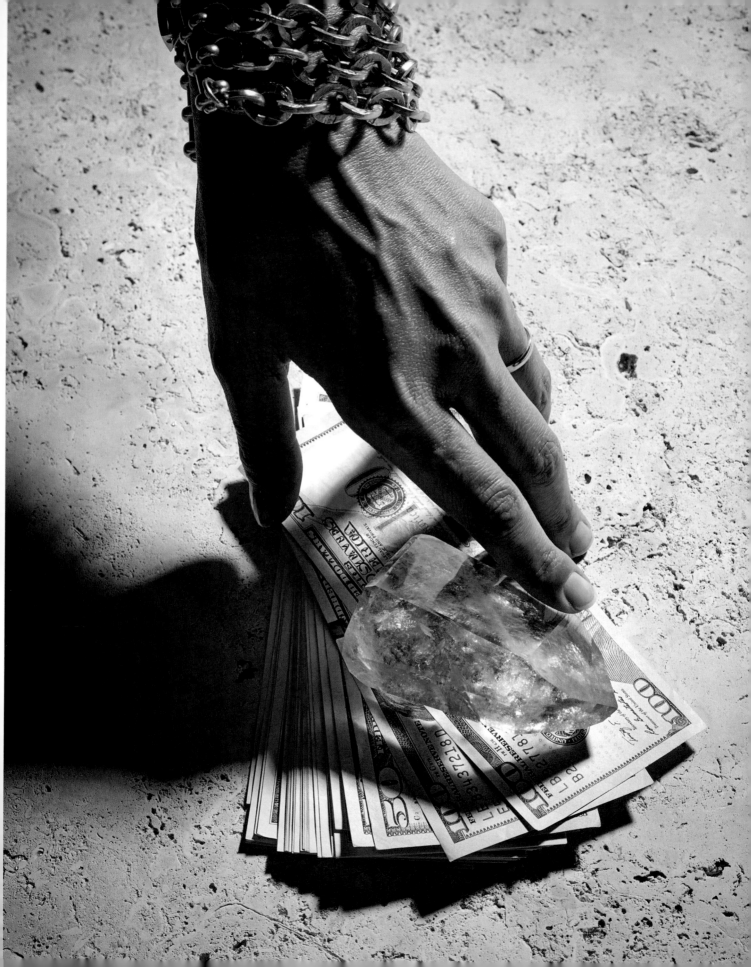

THE ENERGETICS OF MONEY

Money is energy. Simply put. The older and wiser we get, the more we realize that they are one and the same. And, like other forms of energy, there are laws and guiding principles that explain its flow.

As founders of a start-up (and not a tech one) we've had to get used to our share of ebb and flow, otherwise known as instability. Practical methods for managing money are fundamental and essential, but a higher understanding of money's energy allows us to shed limiting beliefs and create true and lasting abundance.

It's important to acknowledge these practices, as money may be the single greatest source of stress and conflict in our world. Befriend money, don't fear for its lack and open yourself up to the possibilities that money may afford you.

We are lucky to have forward-thinking friends and advisors who have shared their visionary-yet-practical techniques for creating abundance. We're still growing (we always will be), but see a profound shift when we practice these principles consistently.

MONEY FLOWS: With the rise of electronic modes of payment, it's easy to see that money can be intangible, a mere idea, yet, very real. If you are in business or simply trying to build a life of abundance, you will undoubtedly experience the highs and lows of cash flow. Recognizing this natural pattern and becoming comfortable with its ways allows you to ride the wave, knowing that, when funds are tight, there will be more to come. Practice faith, and exercise your ability to weather the storm.

KNOW THE WHY: Vision boards, wish lists and unlimited thinking encourage us to shoot for the stars. And, we couldn't agree more, but, as we visualize our wants, we ask ourselves why. When there is a strong mission or a "why" behind any goal, it holds exponential power.

Desires that do not align with the greater good, or your mission, may not be worth the real estate on your vision board. Meditate on what you truly want, and why. When your wants are aligned with your personal North Star, the universe will conspire to help you receive them.

ASK, AND YOU SHALL RECEIVE: Once you're clear about your desires, get in the habit of repeating them. Say them out loud, or write them down. Don't be shy. Ask the universe for what you want. So often, manifesting simply boils down to that.

GIVING THANKS: A universal theme, giving thanks, once again proves its worth. Simply do it. Wake up, and thank the universe for what you have, for the love and riches already in your life and for all that's to come. It works.

SEEING IS BELIEVING: Our manifestation advisor, Lacy, shared this concept with us during a session on prosperity. It's simple but profound. Find a person or cluster of people (we made a composite) who embody the success you desire for yourself. Relate to this person. Make sure that his or her lifestyle or mission is in keeping with yours. It helps if they've faced some of the same challenges that you have. Seeing is believing proves that it's possible. As Dyer says, "You'll see it when you believe it." Done.

TITHING: A long-held practice in almost every faith, tithing works. Technically, tithing is the practice of giving 10 percent of your income to your church or spiritual organization, though many have expanded this to include meaningful charities. Nothing links your personal success to the interest of the greater good so clearly as tithing. Money is energy.

To get started, pick a cause that's important to you. And, if 10 percent terrifies you, start smaller. Try 5 percent, or even less.

NEW MOON JOURNALING

Much like spring itself, the new moon cues new beginnings. Its energies collaborate with our intentions to activate prosperity and change. To harness these energies, pull out your journal and write. The act of putting pen to paper, of clarifying your wants, is all the more powerful when the moon is on your side. Do this on the day of the new moon or in the first few days of its cycle. Consider this a time to clear the debris of the previous moon cycle and to formally invite in a new chapter.

Find a journal you love, and devote this to your moon writings. List your intentions, and be specific. Visualize and elaborate on how you'll feel when your desires are manifested. Go big here, and be grateful for the opportunity to start fresh every month. This monthly check-in with your grandest plans creates accountability and consistency. Stay in touch with your highest self. Or, in the words of Barack Obama, "Show up. Dive in. Stay at it."

HOME

BRANCHING OUT

Bring nature in. Transform your space with the magic of flowering branches. Spring boasts an abundance from quince to cherry blossom to lilac to dogwood and beyond. Shop your local farmer's market or cut some from your yard. A little goes a long way. Cut down to size. Using a hammer, pound the base of each stem, allowing water to penetrate more deeply. Change the water often, and the branches, except the lilacs, can last for up to 2 weeks. Take advantage of spring's bounty, and surround yourself with beauty.

MAKING SPACE

Clear it out. Clean it up. You can't organize clutter, so it's best just to get rid of it. We've all felt the wave of KonMari and its take-no-prisoners approach to clutter. We believe in the power of abundance, but take a detour when it comes to objects in our lives that don't serve us. It's important to make space for what you truly love. Fear or a feeling of lacking often encourages us to hold onto things. Letting go is an act of faith and shows the universe that you are ready to receive.

Be systematic. We like to do this over a series of days, mapping out our homes and tackling a section at a time. You don't have to conquer a whole room in one go. Even clearing a cabinet or drawer or section of your closet has a powerful impact. Make your way around the house donating (or tossing) anything that you don't love. Don't overthink it, just get rid of it.

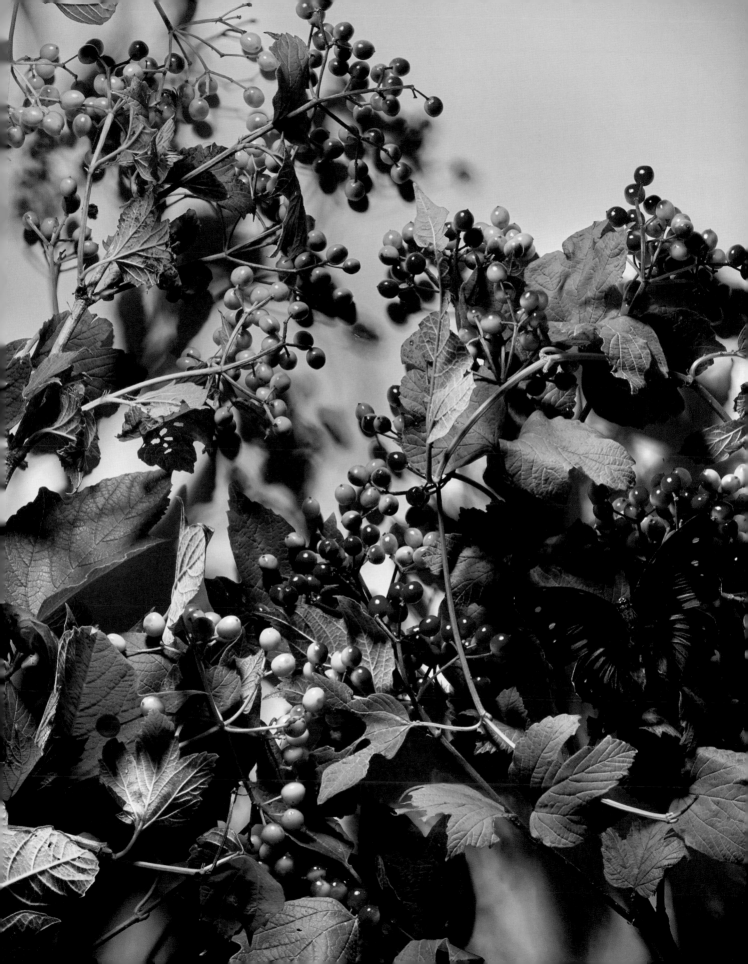

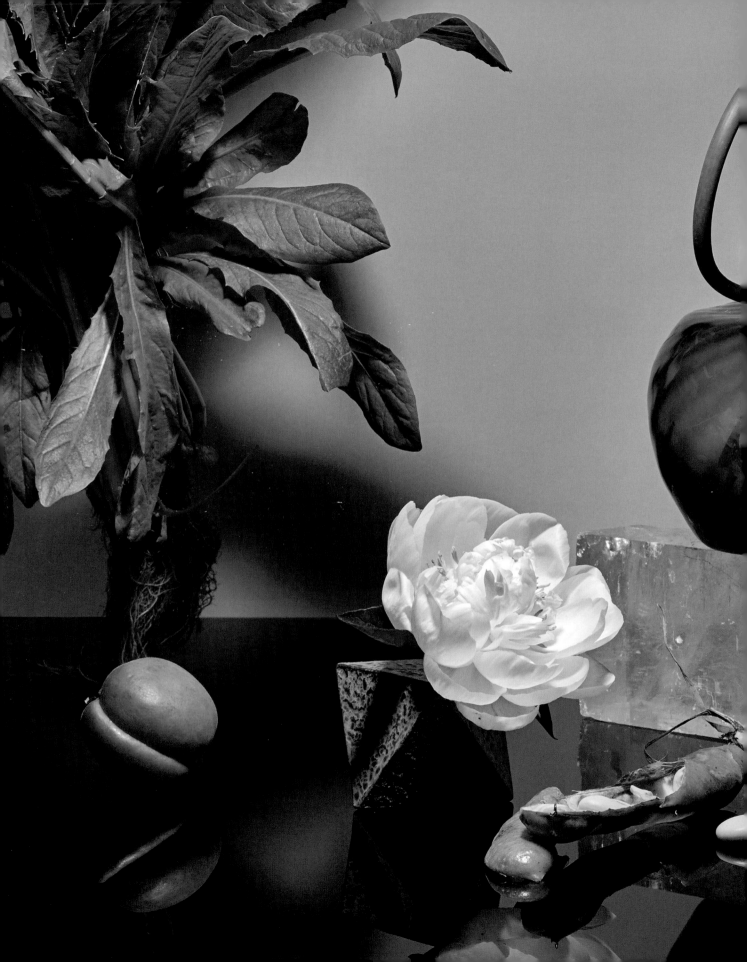

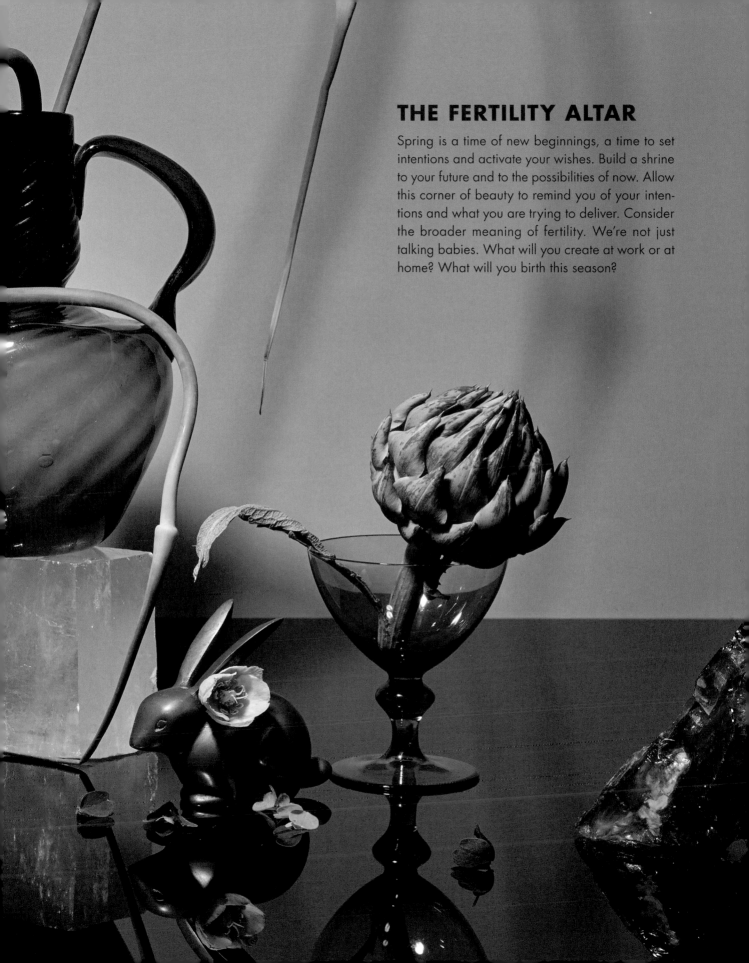

THE FERTILITY ALTAR

Spring is a time of new beginnings, a time to set intentions and activate your wishes. Build a shrine to your future and to the possibilities of now. Allow this corner of beauty to remind you of your intentions and what you are trying to deliver. Consider the broader meaning of fertility. We're not just talking babies. What will you create at work or at home? What will you birth this season?

PART WITH PLASTICS

Act glassy! Become aware of the plastics in your life, and, whenever possible, swap for a healthy and sustainable option. It's an easy upgrade that's good for you, Mother Earth, our children, animals and plants. Skip the plastic water bottles and opt instead for quality filtered water. Take it on the road with you in your own glass water bottle. Invest in a set of glass storage containers. We love a lidded glass pitcher for storing soups and nut and seed milks. You can also recycle glass jars from your groceries. Glass is the enlightened choice. Food tastes better in glass.

A CLEANER CLEAN

Spring cleaning takes on a new meaning when we clean up our cleaning supplies. Most of what we need to keep our homes charged and fresh can be found in the pantry and fridge. Like with our beauty products, we don't focus on the danger of the ingredients in conventional products, but on the power of plants, minerals and Mother Nature.

ALL-PURPOSE CLEANER

This is our favorite cleaner to keep in the cupboard for a healthy, High Vibrational clean. Make a batch of this to have on hand, and your home will be shining all the time.

> **16 ounces hydrogen peroxide**
>
> **⅛ teaspoon mint essential oil**

Combine the ingredients in a glass spray bottle, shake to combine and use.

GLASS CLEANER

This simple-yet-effective cleaner has been used by even the most accomplished cleaners since the beginning of time. As simple as it gets.

> **2 cups filtered water**
>
> **2 tablespoons vinegar**
>
> **1 teaspoon lavender essential oil**

Combine all ingredients in a glass spray bottle, shake to combine and use.

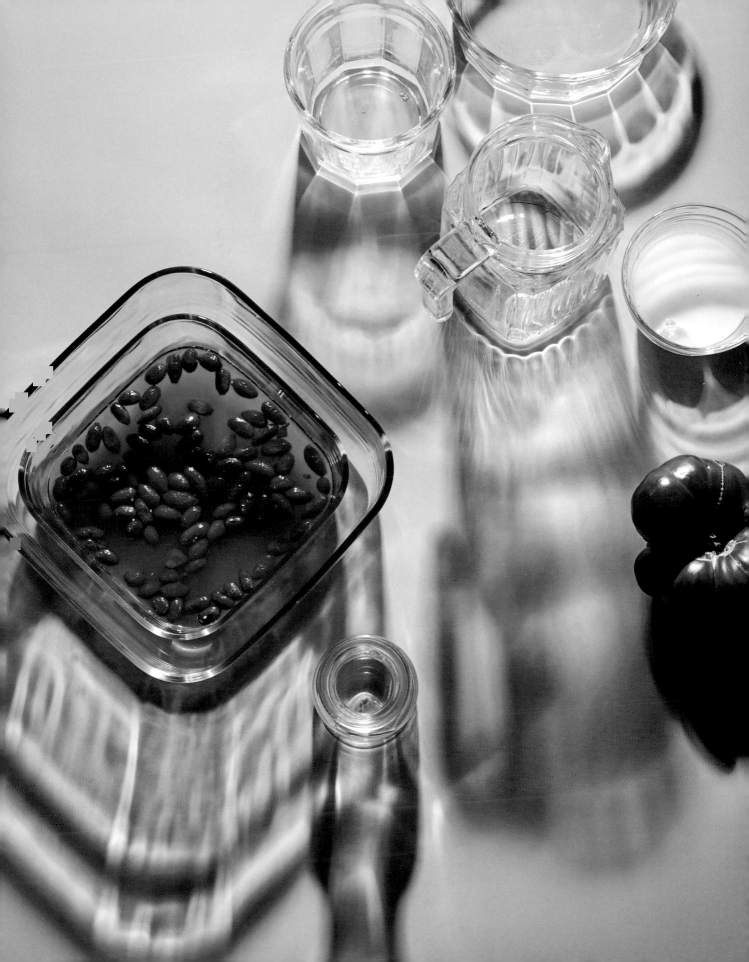

FRIENDS AGAIN

We're something like bears. Laying low for the winter months, spending time at home, seeking solitude. But as the light returns, we come out of "hibernation." We seek companionship and connection. Spending time with friends and loved ones not only feeds our souls, it's nurturing to our bodies and minds, reducing stress and cortisol levels and, some studies show, even increasing longevity. If you shy away from social plans or if, like us, you imagine yourself too busy to socialize, consider this homework. Spend 15 minutes a day reaching out to friends. Make a date with your bestie. Reconnect.

LOVE ANIMALS

Animals make life better. It's as simple as that. Borrow one, adopt one, cuddle with one, or volunteer at your local shelter. Studies show that spending time with these loyal friends can lower blood pressure, reduce stress and increase happiness. And, they just make life better. Consider rescuing your next best friend. That dog or cat (or donkey or horse!) might just rescue you. The Sato Project is a rescue organization that is dear to Kerrilynn's heart. She and her husband, John, were one of the first families to adopt one of their Puerto Rican strays. Beba is now the resident office dog and a spreader of light, even though she can come across a little grumpy. They recently took in another Sato, the 4-pound Ricardo that they call Ricky. Watching his transformation from a scared, and sometimes even aggressive, dog to a relaxed and loving family pet has been enlightening. Ricky and Beba are here to remind us to stay in the present. Love is a powerful and transformative thing.

LEAN ON

This season of reawakening is an ideal time to begin new practices. The inherent optimism of spring gives rise to new habits and encourages positive change. Nothing supports a healthy shift like a friend to lean on. Who in your life will support your shift? And, who can you support? Partnering with a like-minded friend creates a healthy pact. Fortify your mission, and stay on course through accountability with friends. Use technology. Text each other. Create a Google Doc. Do what you need to do. Then, embody the change. There's power in numbers. Find your crew.

A DAY IN THE LIFE:
SPRING FEVER

RISE UP WITH THE LIGHT OF DAY. WARM WEATHER IS EN ROUTE. Visualize your best spring self, and imagine yourself reborn. What do you want to shed? What do you want to embody? Set your intention for your most radiant being. The season of new beginnings is here. This is your time to shine. Start by giving thanks, a morning ritual we do daily. Say it loud, and mean it. There's power in your voice. Then, ask the universe for support. What do you want or need today? Ask for it, and know that it's yours. Get on your mat or your Kundalini sheepskin, and open your portals. Tune in and turn yourself over to 3 minutes of chanting. You are magnificent. Or, sink into a comfortable chair for 20 minutes of transcendental meditation. Let yourself go deep. Feel the energy rise as you make your way to the kitchen, the land of nourishment. Serve yourself a big glass of filtered water. Add fresh lemon or ACV, and drink up. Don't forget your probiotics. Make a heart-opening tonic, and welcome the day. Then, find your journal and find your center. Write it out. Anything and everything that comes to mind. Don't edit. Don't judge. Just write. Head to the park to get your sweat on. Meet a friend, meet a lover or take your dog out. Run, jump and engage with the power of your body. Try intervals, and find your edge. Head home for a shower and a nourishing meal. A matcha pudding or a smoothie or the Far Out Temple Bowl (page 56) are all on offer. Pick your potion. Then, indulge in a day of beauty. Head out for a facial or infrared sauna, or lavish yourself at home. A day of dry brushing, baths and replenishing masks electrifies you in every way. Radiate. Turn on the Hifi, pull out your favorite book, and let yourself be inspired. Creativity cures. Feed your brain. Drink a green juice, and head to the kitchen to prepare a feast for your friends. Try a board with cheese made from plants, crackers made from seeds and the Begin Again Hummus (page 64). This is dinner reinvented. Pour pine pollen fizzes for your crew, and know that tomorrow you'll feel great. Stand in the light. Start a game of charades. Engage your mind and body. They work better together. Goodnight kisses all around. Love abounds where deep health thrives. Thank the day for all it has offered. Tomorrow will shine.

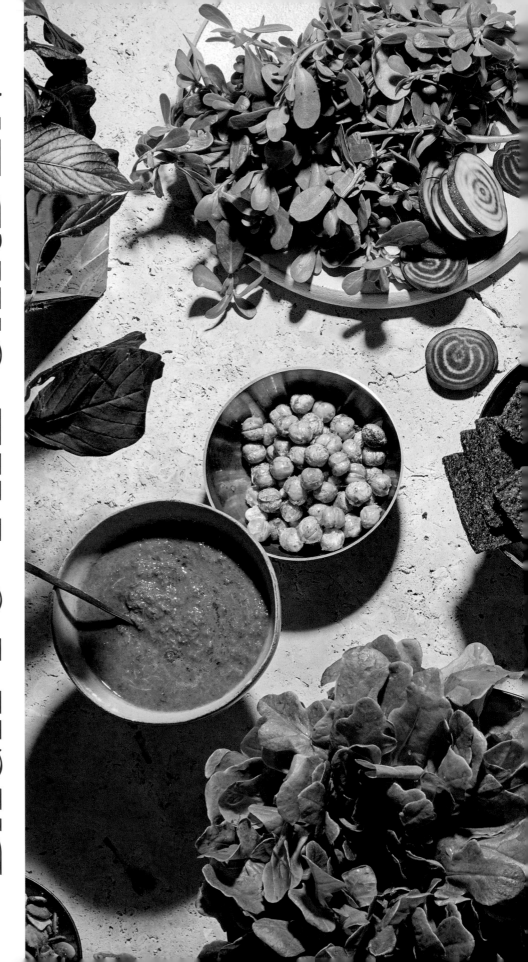

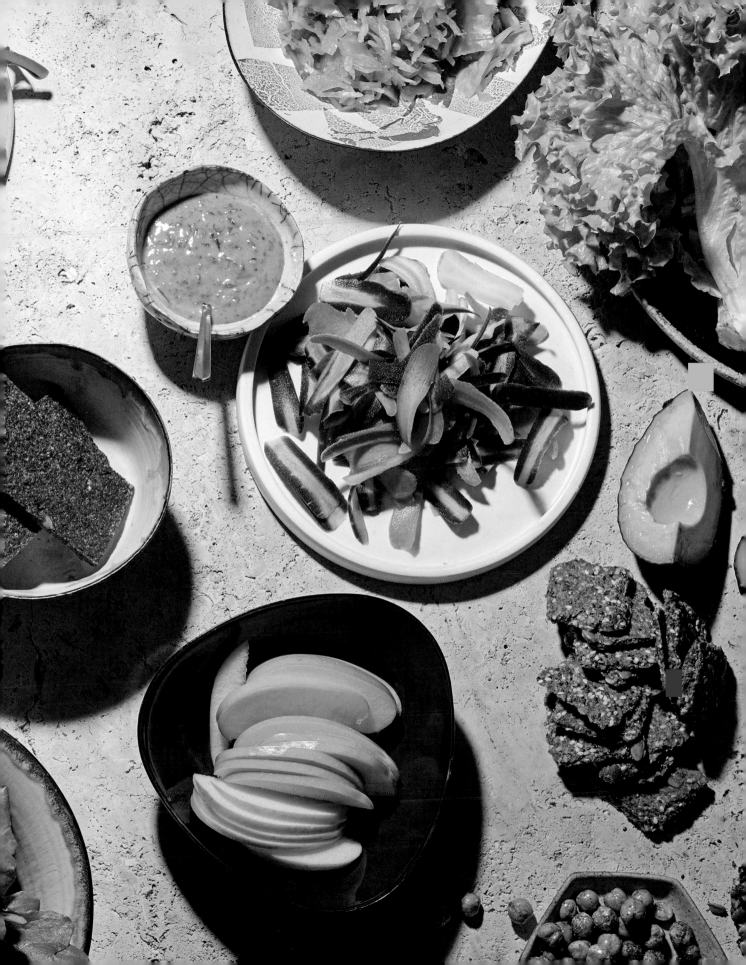

SHARE THE LOVE:
HIPPIE SALAD NIGHT

Cindy is infamous for her inclusive and feel-good gatherings, and Hippie Salad Night is legend. Based on the salad bars of our youth and the dream of a big and magical California-style bowl, Hippie Salad Night presents an altar of greens, dressings and delicious toppings, and the chance to show off a collection of beautiful dishes.

And, her foodie friends don't mind at all. Everyone loves to build, create and flaunt their own combos. And, since guests create their own meals, it's also a great party for anyone with allergies and diet restrictions.

Not for the faint of heart, this dinner requires more than its share of shopping and prep, but there's little to cook and most can be done in advance. And, that adds up to more time spent with friends. Grab a bowl, and be here now.

HERE'S HOW TO DO IT: Fill two large bowls, the biggest you have, with washed and dried lettuces. We like to offer one light and bright, like Boston or Bibb, and one darker variety like massaged kale or arugula. Then, set out your toppings. Pick as many as you can from our list below and add your own as well. Abundance is key! Create the salad bar of your dreams, and think in terms of balanced tastes, something sweet and something salty. Add a board of gluten-free bread and crackers with a side of ghee or Cashew Quark (see page 253) and a pretty little dish of Himalayan pink salt. This is comfort food after all.

Apples, sliced finely and soaked in fresh lemon juice	Sprouts and microgreens	Tomatoes	Nutritional yeast
Pepitas, toasted (or Berbere, page 267)	Steamed broccoli	Shredded cabbage	Cooked brown rice, millet or quinoa
Tamari almonds (page 49)	Hemp seeds	Carrot Salad (opposite)	Cashew Quark (page 253)
	Sunflower seeds	Avocados	So-Many-Seeds Crackers (page 271)
	Sauerkraut	Roasted Chickpea Croutons (opposite)	
	Dulse flakes		

Here are the perfect toppings to your salads. Make sure your salad bar has good-quality olive oil and fresh lemons, as well as these vibrant dressings.

LSD (opposite)	Green Goddess Tahini (page 42)	Miso Dressing (page 42)

CARROT SALAD

We make this a lot and store it in the fridge to add to weeknight dinner bowls.

6 big carrots, trimmed and grated

Big pinch of Himalayan pink salt

1 cup pepitas, soaked and dehydrated or toasted

Olive oil

Juice of 1 lemon, or to taste

½ cup finely chopped chives

Add the carrots, salt and seeds to a large mixing bowl. Dress with oil and lemon, and toss to combine thoroughly. Add the chives and toss once more.

ROASTED CHICKPEA CROUTONS

3 cups cooked chickpeas or 2 (15-ounce) cans chickpeas

Coconut oil, to taste

Big pinch of Himalayan pink salt

2 tablespoons Berbere (page 267) or 1 tablespoon each turmeric, ground ginger and ground black pepper

Preheat the oven to 400°F. Toss the chickpeas in a large mixing bowl with oil, the salt and spices. Spread onto a parchment-lined baking sheet and roast for 20 to 30 minutes. Remove from the oven and let cool. Store in the refrigerator and use within a week.

LSD

Based on the famous lemon-sesame dressing from the now closed Cabbagetown Cafe, Ithaca's other vegetarian restaurant.

¼ cup sesame seeds, toasted

1 cup olive oil

Juice of 2 lemons

2 tablespoons apple cider vinegar

1 tablespoon tamari

1 to 2 scallions, coarsely chopped

Handful of chives, coarsely chopped

Handful of parsley leaves and stems, coarsely chopped

Handful of basil leaves

Big pinch of Himalayan pink salt

½ teaspoon mustard powder

Place all ingredients into a blender and blend until smooth. Trip out.

GREEN GODDESS TAHINI

A classic dressing with a new twist. The radish or scallion microgreens will add bite! This dressing will thicken in the fridge, so don't worry if you overthin it a bit.

1 cup tahini

Juice of 2 lemons or a few

¼ tablespoon apple cider vinegar

1 clove garlic

Big pinch of Himalayan pink salt

½ cup basil leaves, coarsely chopped

½ cup parsley leaves

½ cup chives, coarsely chopped

¼ cup radish or scallion microgreens (optional)

Filtered water

Place all ingredients except for water in a high-speed blender and blend until the herbs are thoroughly blended. With motor on low speed, slowly drizzle in filtered water until the dressing reaches the desired consistency. Alternatively, you can finely chop the ingredients by hand, and use a hand whisk to blend the dressing.

MISO DRESSING

A nice Asian-inspired dressing that goes well with every salad. Use the miso of your choice for this sure-to-please favorite.

4 tablespoons miso

Juice of 2 or 3 lemons or ¼ cup apple cider vinegar

2 tablespoons dark sesame oil

1 (1-inch) piece of ginger, peeled and grated

¾ cup olive or coconut oil

½ cup filtered water

In a small bowl, whisk together the miso, lemon juice or vinegar, sesame oil and ginger. Slowly add the olive or coconut oil, whisking as you go. Then, slowly drizzle in the water until the dressing is pourable. You can also do this in a blender, adding the oil and water with the blender on low speed.

Inspired by our friends at By Chloe, these savory noodles marry comfort and health. A match made in heaven. We like to serve this on top of a bed of fresh spring greens with a heaping forkful of fermented vegetables and a sprinkling of sprouted pumpkin seeds.

PACIFIC DREAM KELP NOODLES

½ cup raw cashews

Juice from ½ lime

¼ teaspoon Himalayan pink salt

½ teaspoon coconut aminos or tamari

3 tablespoons water or brewed matcha

½ teaspoon organic matcha powder

6 ounces kelp noodles

Handful of chopped chives or cilantro, for serving (optional)

Add the cashews, lime juice, salt, coconut aminos or tamari, water or matcha and matcha powder to a food processor and blend until easily pourable. Rinse the noodles and, using kitchen shears, cut them to the desired length. Pour the matcha sauce over the noodles and toss to coat. Serve with the chives or cilantro, if using.

SERVES 2

COCONUT AMINOS

Put down the soy sauce and grab the coconut aminos. Made from just tree sap and salt, this stand-in for soy sauce is one of our favorite swaps in the High Vibrational kitchen. With a slightly sweeter flavor than traditional soy sauce, this condiment lends itself well to breakfast, lunch and dinner. Known to strengthen the immune system, protect the heart and support mental health, this is a staple that we never go without. Store it in the fridge.

One of our favorite superfruits of all is the tangy, tart and sweet golden-berry. They look like a little orange cherry tomato with a papery case like a tomatillo, but we're equal fans of the dried variety, available year-round at health food stores. Golden Hour Granola greets the morning with all the brightness of this magical, mystical, underused fruit. Get to know the goldenberry.

GOLDEN HOUR GRANOLA

2 cups gluten-free oats

1½ cup millet seeds

¾ cup sunflower seeds

¾ cup pumpkin seeds

1 cup unsweetened coconut flakes

1 ripe banana, chopped

½ cup coconut oil

¼ cup + 1 tablespoon maple syrup

1 teaspoon vanilla extract (or ½ vanilla bean)

1 teaspoon turmeric

½ teaspoon ground ginger

½ teaspoon Himalayan pink salt

1 cup fresh or dried goldenberries

Preheat the oven to 300°F.

In a large mixing bowl, combine the oats, millet seeds, sunflower seeds, pumpkin seeds and coconut flakes. Mix well and set aside.

In a medium saucepan over medium heat, gently warm the banana, oil, syrup, vanilla, turmeric, ginger and salt. Cook for about 5 minutes in order for the flavors to meld together. Carefully transfer this to a food processor and process until the banana is pureed. Pour into the seed mixture and stir until well-combined. Spread out on a parchment-lined baking sheet and cook for 30 minutes, stirring every 10 minutes, until golden brown and crispy. When cool enough to handle, transfer to a large mixing bowl and toss in the goldenberries.

NOTE: Alternatively, you can dehydrate this at 105° to 115°F for 18 to 24 hours.

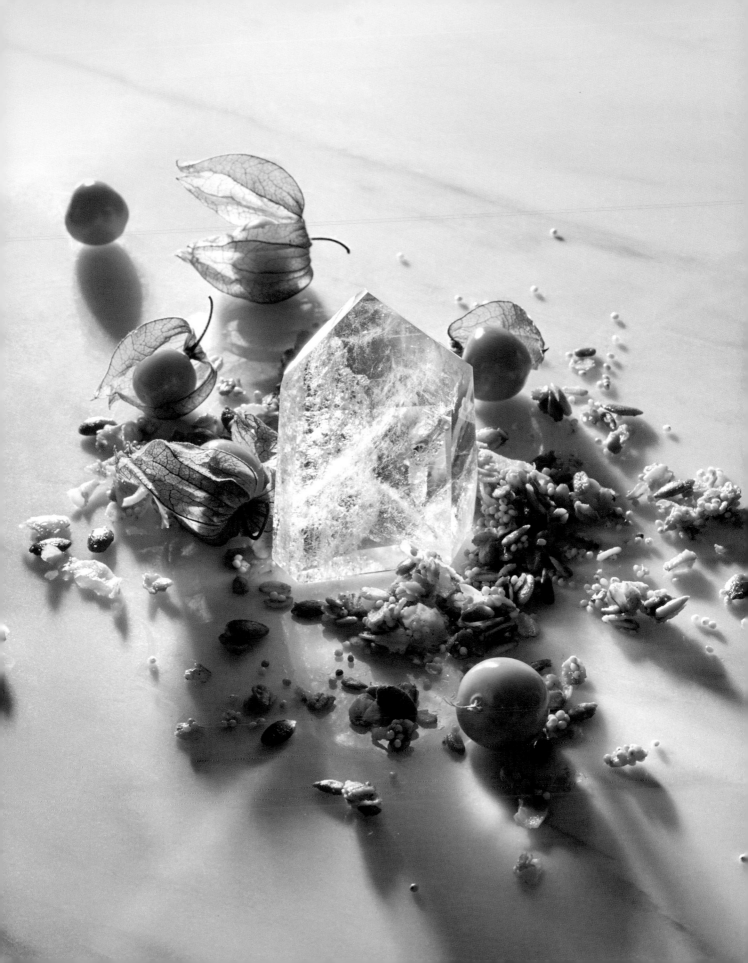

A true *farinata* is made from only chickpea flour, oil and water, but we're not known for our minimalist ways. And, where we see a culinary canvas, we add green. Cindy is known for her huge and satisfying dinner salads, and, lately, she's been topping it off with a slice of this. An uplevel that's welcome to all. *Buongiorno e buon appetito.*

GREEN EARTH *FARINATA*

1½ cups chickpea flour

2 cups filtered water

Zest of 1 lemon

1 tablespoon Himalayan pink salt

2 cups baby or mature spinach

1 bunch parsley

1 cup mint leaves

3 to 4 cloves garlic

Coconut oil

VINAIGRETTE

½ shallot, minced

1 teaspoon lemon juice

1 teaspoon ume plum vinegar or apple cider vinegar

½ teaspoon honey or coconut sugar (optional)

½ teaspoon Dijon mustard

½ cup olive oil

⅛ teaspoon Himalayan pink salt

SALAD

2 cups baby spring greens

2 radishes, sliced thin

1 cup fresh English peas, blanched

¼ cup Botija olives, halved

Herbs

Combine the flour, water, lemon zest and 1½ teaspoons of the salt in a large bowl and let it rest for at least an hour. Meanwhile, bring about 8 cups water to a boil in a large saucepan. Make sure to have an ice bath ready nearby. In stages, carefully drop in all of the greens and cook them until they become bright green. Using a slotted spatula, quickly transfer them to the ice bath. Add the garlic to the saucepan, and cook for 1 to 2 minutes, or until softened. Drain the greens and the garlic from the ice bath and squeeze out any excess moisture with an absorbent dish towel. Transfer to a food processor and pulse a few times to break down the greens. Add the reserved chickpea batter and process until you have a bright green batter, about 1 minute. Set aside.

To make the vinaigrette: Place the shallot, lemon juice, vinegar, honey or coconut sugar (if using) and mustard into a small mixing bowl. Whisk to combine. Slowly pour in the oil while continuing to whisk. Sprinkle in the salt. Set aside.

To cook the farinata: Heat up a large skillet over medium-high heat. Add 1 teaspoon coconut oil. Allow the oil to heat up for 15 to 30 seconds. Tilt the pan so that the oil covers the entire surface and immediately drop about ¼ of the batter into the skillet. Tilt and rotate the pan to form a "pancake." Then, allow it to cook until the edges begin to bubble and the bottom releases. With a spatula, flip the pancake in half to form a half-moon shape. Continue to cook this for about a minute longer. Remove from the pan and repeat with the remaining batter.

To make the salad: In a medium mixing bowl, toss the greens, radishes, peas, olives, herbs and vinaigrette together. Divide the salad evenly on top of the pancakes right before serving.

SERVES 4

These creamy, dense and delicious muffins are inspired by our love for overnight oats and berry muffins made from them. Swap your mason jar for a muffin tin and take in the same raw power. Delicious cold with a cup of hot tea. Breakfast just got better.

BERRY BOMBES

2 cups gluten-free rolled oats

2 cups nut or seed milk

¼ cup unsweetened coconut flakes

¼ cup nut or seed butter

1 tablespoon chia seeds

1 tablespoon flaxseeds, ground

2 tablespoons maple syrup

1 teaspoon cinnamon

½ teaspoon Himalayan pink salt

½ cup mixed dried berries (goji, mulberries, goldenberries)

Add the oats, milk, coconut, nut butter, chia seeds, flaxseeds, syrup, cinnamon and salt into a food processor and process until well combined. Toss in the berries and pulse a few times to incorporate. Form balls using about ¼ cup of batter each. Place in a storage container and refrigerate overnight to enjoy the following day.

MAKES 12

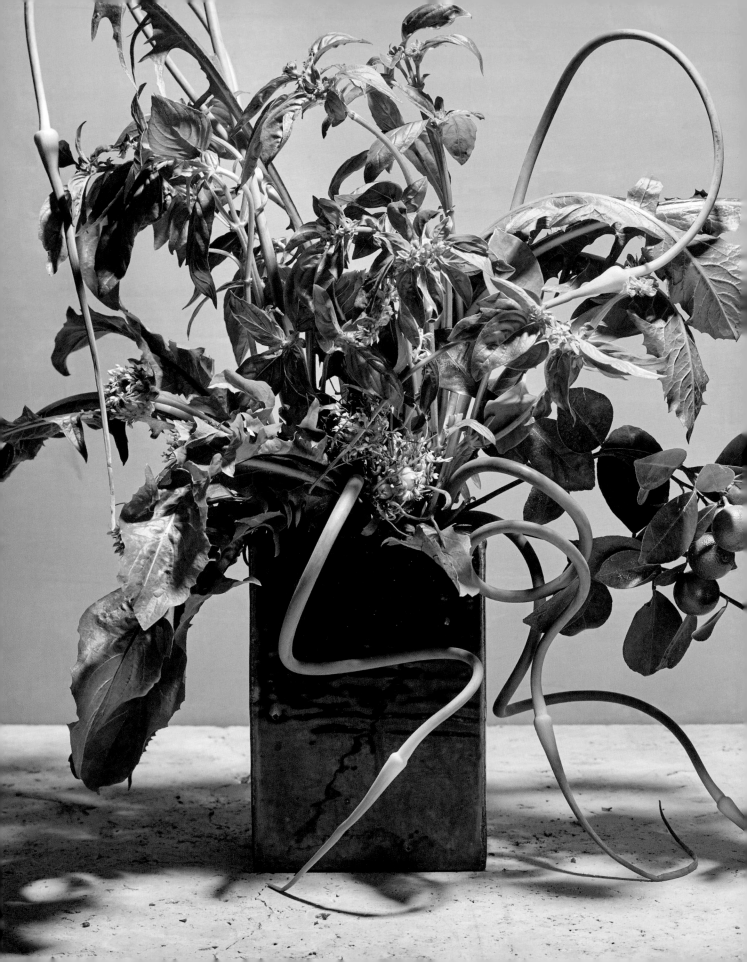

Spring brings a bounty of tonifying and cleansing herbs, and dandelion and nettle are two of the greats. Up your intake of these powerhouse greens by blending them into a simple pesto. Serve over raw or blanched zucchini noodles for a familiar and much-loved dish with hidden health benefits to boot. Tone up your day.

TONIC YOUTH PESTO

3 cups basil leaves

1 cup dandelion and/or nettle leaves

⅔ cup pumpkin seeds, toasted

⅓ cup hemp seeds

1 small garlic clove, chopped

2 tablespoons tamari

¼ teaspoon salt

3 tablespoons olive oil

1 tablespoon + 1 teaspoon fresh lemon juice

In a food processor, combine the basil, dandelion and/or nettle, pumpkin seeds, hemp seeds, garlic, tamari, and salt. Process until well-combined. While the machine is running, slowly pour in the oil. When ready to serve, stir in the lemon juice to keep the sauce green and vibrant.

MAKES 1½ CUPS

TAMARI

As you convert your kitchen to a place free from gluten and rich in nuanced and balanced flavors, you'll swap your standard soy sauce for this High Vibrational Japanese version. Unlike common soy sauce, tamari is made without wheat. (Double check the package, as some tamaris do contain small amounts of wheat.) And, while both are made from fermented soy beans, tamari is a more-balanced, rich and delicate ingredient. Look for organic and non-GMO. Then, get right at it with a homemade batch of Tamari almonds. On a sheet pan, simply oven-roast the almonds for 20 minutes at 300°F. Remove and toss with a few spoonfuls of tamari. Then, return to the oven for 5 minutes more. We love these added to salads or dragon bowls.

Seasonal greens pack more than their share of alkalizing phytonutrients and healthy fiber. At CAP Beauty, we look for ways to add heft to our salads to create more satisfying meals from our go-to greens. We serve these grain-free crepes as the base for a big plate of greens that satisfies even our hungriest dinner dates.

MOUNTAIN HIGH CHICKPEA CREPES

1 bunch seasonal greens, such as sorrel, dandelion, nettles

2 heads baby lettuce

1 fennel bulb, thinly sliced

1 teaspoon chopped tarragon

1 teaspoon chopped chives

1 tablespoon raw sprouted pumpkin seeds

8 green olives, pitted and sliced

Juice of ½ lemon

Olive oil, to taste

Flaky sea salt, to taste

CREPES

1 cup sprouted chickpea flour

1 tablespoon olive or coconut oil, plus more for pan

1 cup filtered water

½ teaspoon salt

Pumpkin seed butter, coconut mayonnaise or tahini dressing

Black pepper, to taste

Start by assembling the salad. (You can substitute any salad recipe you love.) When the crepes are hot, you'll want to eat them right away! Place the greens, lettuces, fennel, tarragon, chives, pumpkin seeds and olives in a deep salad bowl. Dress generously with the lemon juice, oil and salt. Set aside.

To make the crepes: Add the flour, oil, water and salt to a medium mixing bowl and whisk until blended. Heat a nonstick skillet or crepe pan over medium high heat. Add oil to coat. When the oil is hot, pour ¼ to ½ cup of batter into the pan and gently swirl the pan to spread the batter evenly. Watch carefully, and when the top begins to bubble and the underside is a light golden brown, flip the crepe to cook the other side for about a minute. Transfer to a plate and repeat with the remaining batter.

To serve, place a crepe on each plate, spread with a coating of pumpkin seed butter, coconut mayo or tahini and pile high with salad greens. Keep extras in a warm oven.

SERVES 4

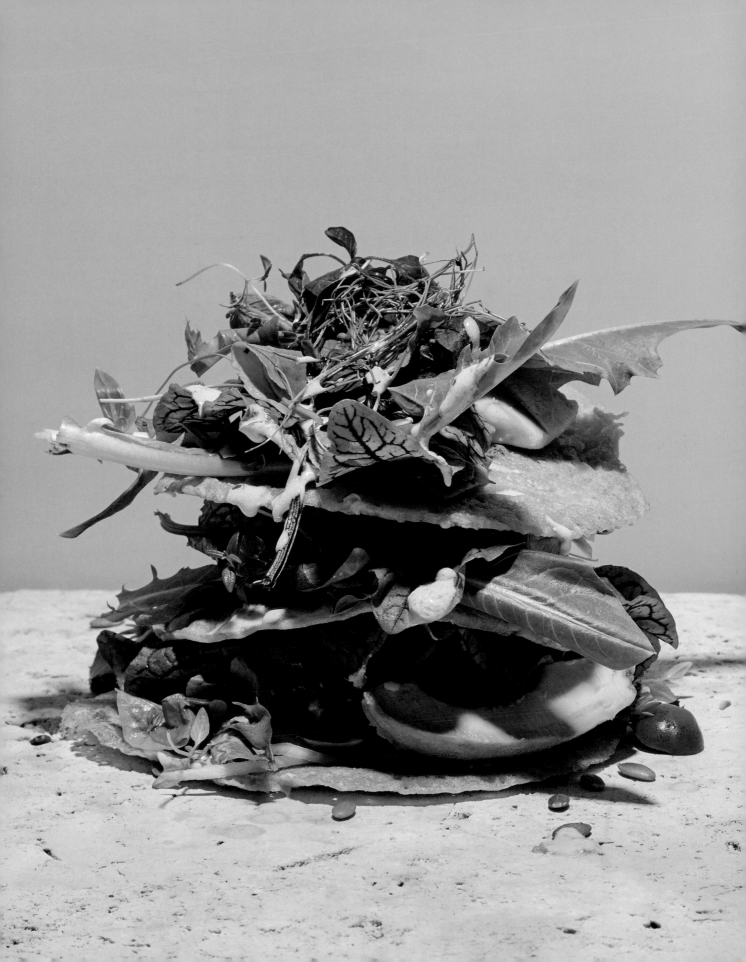

We lovingly refer to this as "the Pizza Hut salad" as it reminds us of a bottomless crisp and addictive salad more likely to be served in a chain restaurant than a health food hub. Fortunately, our version is filled with only healthful and High Vibe ingredients, so dig in and fly high.

HOLY SMOKE CAESAR

2 heads romaine hearts

½ cucumber, thinly sliced

½ zucchini, grated

½ avocado, pitted and sliced

¼ cup botija olives or dried and cured black olives

¼ cup sprouted and roasted sunflower seeds

½ cup sunflower sprouts

DRESSING
¼ cup tahini

Juice from ½ lemon

1 teaspoon liquid aminos or tamari

1 tablespoon Taste of Tomoko (page 266)

2 tablespoons water or olive oil, plus more as needed

Tear the romaine into manageable pieces, add to your favorite big salad bowl, and top with all other salad ingredients.

To make the dressing: Add the tahini, lemon juice, liquid aminos or tamari and Tomoko spices to a bowl or blender. Whisk or blend until combined. Continue mixing and slowly add the water or oil until it reaches the desired consistency (we like it pretty thick). Toss with the salad, adding a little at a time, until evenly coated. (Refrigerate any leftover dressing, to enjoy later.)

SERVES 2 AS A MAIN DISH OR 4 AS A SIDE DISH

Inspired by one of our favorite restaurants, New York City's EN Japanese Brasserie, this simple yet sophisticated Japanese take on crudité is our favorite opener for a dinner party. Perfectly steamed vegetables paired with a miso dipping sauce sets the tone for a Japanese feast. Can you tell how much we love Japan yet?

SHRINE ON: JAPANESE VEGETABLES WITH MISO DIPPING SAUCE

4 cups mixed herbs

1 clove garlic, chopped

1 small avocado

¼ cup tahini

1 tablespoon chickpea miso

Juice of 1 lemon

¼ cup filtered water, plus more as needed

Assorted steamed spring vegetables (snow or sugar snap peas, English peas, radishes, baby carrots, spring greens, asparagus)

1 to 1½ cups Nefertiti Spice Shake (page 265)

½ cup mixed herbs, leaves only

Extra-virgin olive oil

Himalayan pink salt, to taste

Fill a medium saucepan with water and place it over high heat. While the water comes to a boil, prepare an ice bath. Once the water boils, drop in the herbs to blanch. Keep them in there for about 15 seconds, or until they become bright green, then remove and plunge them into the ice bath. After 5 minutes or so, remove them from the ice bath and place them on an absorbent kitchen towel, squeezing out any excess moisture. Transfer them to a high-speed blender, add the garlic, avocado, tahini, miso, lemon juice and water, and blend until well-combined. Add more water, if necessary.

Arrange the vegetables on a platter and spoon the herb puree liberally over the top. Sprinkle on the Nefertiti Spice Shake and the herb leaves. Finish with a drizzle of olive oil and some Himalayan salt.

SERVES 4

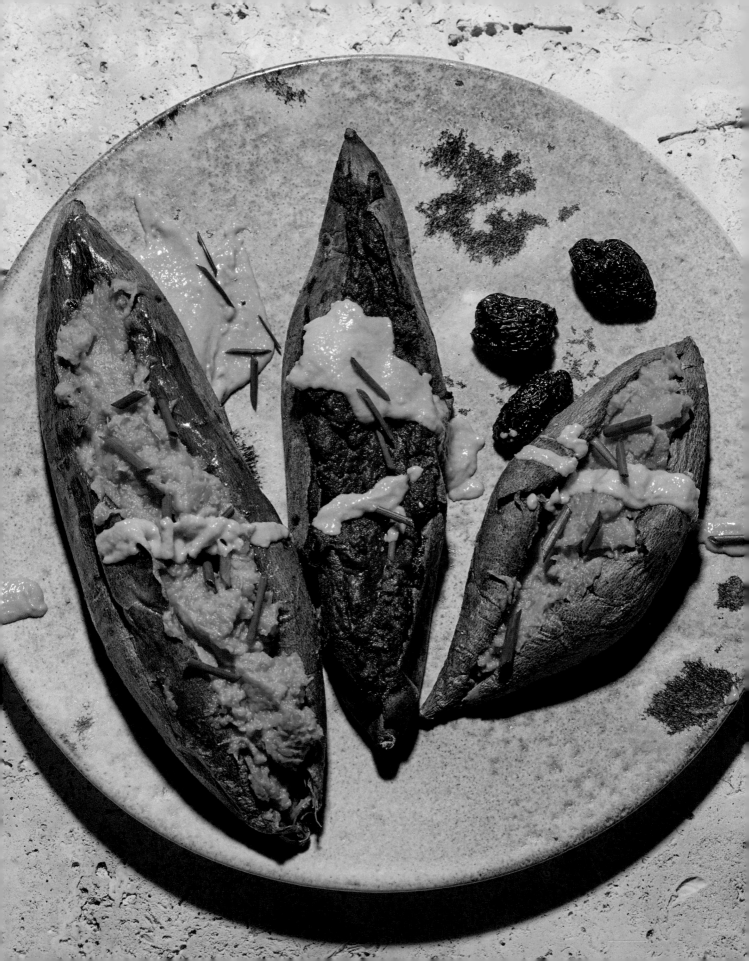

When comfort calls, we listen. This easy weeknight dinner is made complete with a side of greens and a binge-worthy TV show. Or, serve them at a party with bowls of toppings, and welcome your friends to the cult.

TWICE AS NICE STUFFED SWEET POTATOES

4 small to medium sweet potatoes

2 tablespoons coconut oil

½ cup Cashew Quark (page 253)

3 tablespoons nutritional yeast

1 tablespoon chopped chives

1 teaspoon Himalayan pink salt

1 teaspoon ground black pepper

TOPPINGS

Green Goddess Tahini (page 42)

Chopped black olives

Sauerkraut

Chopped chives

Salt and ground black pepper

Sprouted sunflower seeds

Preheat the oven to 350°F. Clean the sweet potatoes and puncture the skin a few times with a fork. Wrap individually in foil, and bake for 35 minutes, or until the potatoes feel soft to the touch. Remove from the oven and let stand until just cool enough to handle.

Unwrap and cut each potato in half lengthwise. Scoop out the flesh, reserving the skins, and add to a large mixing bowl along with the oil, cashew quark, yeast, chives, salt and pepper. Whisk or beat vigorously with a fork until combined. Lay the skins out on a cookie sheet and stuff each with the sweet potato mixture. Broil until the tops are lightly browned. Top with any and all of the toppings.

SERVES 4 AS A MAIN DISH OR 8 AS A SIDE DISH

NOTE: You can stuff the potatoes up to a day ahead and refrigerate until ready to serve. Bake the stuffed potatoes to warm them through before setting them under the broiler.

Channel your inner monk and seek peace (and sustenance!) with this temple worthy meal. The electric greens sit atop forbidden black rice for a psychedelic delicacy. Turn on, tune in and drop out.

FAR OUT TEMPLE BOWL

⅛ teaspoon coriander seeds

1 can coconut milk, unshaken

½ medium yellow onion, thinly sliced

1 (3-inch) knob of ginger, sliced

1 small serrano pepper, halved and sliced

1 tablespoon tamari or coconut aminos

1 tablespoon Taste of Tomoko (page 266)

2 tablespoons of your favorite curry

2 large bunches spinach

Juice of 1 lime

¼ cup cilantro leaves, coarsely chopped

Cooked black rice

Kimchi or fermented red cabbage

Toast the coriander seeds in a dry skillet over medium heat until they pop. Pay close attention so they don't burn. Set aside.

Without shaking, open the coconut milk and scoop out a large spoonful of the thick cream on top, reserving the rest. Place the coconut cream in a heavy bottomed pan or Dutch oven and heat over medium heat. Sauté the onion, ginger and pepper in the cream until translucent. Add the tamari or coconut aminos, Taste of Tomoko, favorite curry and toasted coriander seeds, stirring to coat. Add the remaining coconut milk and bring to a very low simmer. Add the spinach and let it wilt. Stir well, drizzle generously with lime juice and cilantro and serve on top of the rice with a big side of the kimchi or cabbage.

SERVES 2

When salty calls, we answer with a great big bowl of greens laced with the oceanic and umami flavors of seaweed. Tomatoes sweeten the deal, while big slices of avocado and nutty hemp seeds lend their magic. You can toss with a bit of oil, but it's also great without. A perfectly balanced bowl to mineralize and revitalize. Make it big. Eat it all. Answer the call. You can go for darker leafy greens or for fresher young lettuces like little gems or Bibb. Microgreens can be spicy or mild. Use what you love. For the pepitas, use our recipe on page 115, or we love the ones from Sprouties or Moon Juice.

MINERALIZE ME SALAD

2 to 4 cups mixed spring lettuces and sprouts or microgreens

Juice of ½ a lemon or 1 lime

Avocado or olive oil, to taste (optional)

Handful of dried dulse, shells and stones removed

Big handful of cherry tomatoes, halved

¼ to ½ avocado, pitted and sliced or diced

2 heaping tablespoons hemp seeds

2 tablespoons John's Bright, Light Pepitas (page 115), other seasoned pepitas, or crumbled raw crackers

Place the lettuces and sprouts or microgreens in your favorite big salad bowl, tearing any large pieces. Toss with the lemon or lime juice and oil (if using). Add the dulse and tomatoes and continue to toss. Top with the avocado, hemp seeds and pepitas or crackers. Eat it straight from the bowl and feel yourself come alive.

SERVES 1 OR 2

The classic cheese board meets its High Vibration makeover. You can ditch the dairy and still enjoy all of the ceremony and style of a beautifully turned-out board. Swap cow-, goat-, or sheep-milk cheeses for pungent and mild cheeses made from fermented nut and seed milks. Add raw crackers and crudité, dehydrated fruits like persimmons or apples and spice blends or sauces to top it off. Impress your guests or play hostess to yourself. Cheers, dears.

THE SPRING BOARD

Sunflower Seed Chèvre (page 60)

Seeded Brie (page 60)

Cashew Quark (page 253)

Berbere (page 267)

So-Many-Seeds Crackers (page 271)

A Sour Brown Bread (page 269)

Dried fruit of choice (pineapple, papaya, persimmons, apples)

Endive

Radishes

Nut or seed mix of choice

On your favorite wooden board, lay out the cheeses, breads and bowls of crackers and other sides. Have fun, get messy and go for the unexpected. Consider this your High Vibe altar to friends and good living.

SERVES 4 TO 6

RECIPE CONTINUES

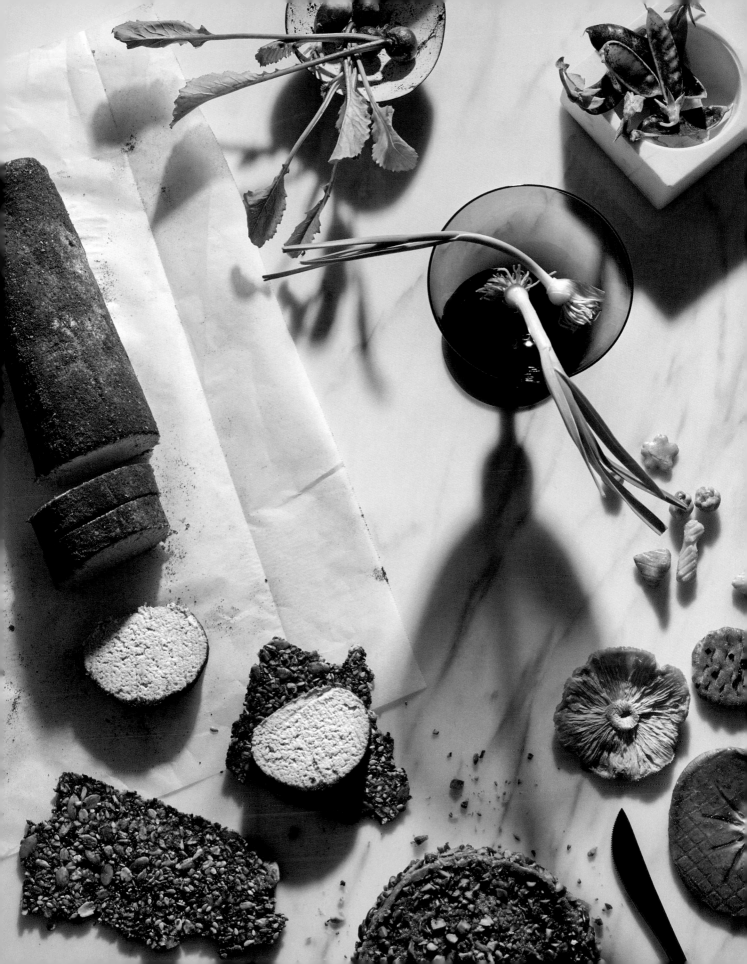

SUNFLOWER SEED CHÈVRE

2 cups raw sunflower seeds, soaked for 6 to 8 hours

2 vegan probiotic capsules or ¼ cup rejuvelac

3 tablespoons filtered water

½ teaspoon Himalayan pink salt

1 to 2 teaspoons fresh lemon juice

Handful of chopped herbs (optional)

Drain the seeds and place them in a high-speed blender with the probiotics or rejuvelac and water. Blend on high until smooth. Place in a bowl covered with cheesecloth and set on your counter for 24 to 36 hours. Alternatively, you can place it in the dehydrator on the lowest setting for 12 to 18 hours. Once fermented to your liking, transfer to a medium bowl and stir in the salt and lemon juice. Transfer to a sheet of parchment and roll into a log shape using cheesecloth. Refrigerate for at least 8 hours. Right before serving, coat the log with herbs, if using. Place the herbs on a flat surface and roll the log in the herbs until they adhere.

MAKES 1 LOG OR 1 CUP

SEEDED BRIE

1 cup pumpkin seeds, soaked for 8 hours

1 cup sunflower seeds, soaked for 8 hours

2 vegan probiotic capsules

3 tablespoons filtered water

2 tablespoons nutritional yeast

½ teaspoon Himalayan pink salt

1 to 2 teaspoons fresh lemon juice

Drain the seeds and place them in a high-speed blender with the probiotics and water. Blend on high until smooth. Place in a bowl covered with cheesecloth and set on your counter for 24 to 36 hours. Alternatively, you can place it in the dehydrator on the lowest setting for 12 to 18 hours. Once fermented to your liking, transfer to a medium bowl and stir in the yeast, salt and lemon juice. Transfer to a small parchment-lined springform pan or ring mold. Refrigerate for 4 hours to set. Carefully transfer the cheese and parchment from the pan onto a dehydrator sheet. Dehydrate at 145°F for 1 hour, reduce the heat to the lowest setting and continue to heat for 24 to 36 hours or until the cheese has developed a nice rind.

MAKES 1 ROUND OR 1 CUP

Inspired by the doyenne of the Ithaca, New York, vegetarian cooking scene, Mollie Katzen, this dish is on constant rotation in our homes. Broccoli sits amongst a tangle of kelp noodles spiked with ginger and tamari and proves, once again, that Ithaca is gorges.

OCEAN OISHII NOODLES

1 package kelp noodles

2 cups broccoli florets, chopped

1 teaspoon freshly grated ginger

4 umeboshi plums, chopped

4 cups filtered water

4 teaspoons good quality genmaicha

4 teaspoons coconut aminos or tamari

2 sheets toasted nori, cut into small pieces

4 teaspoons Holy Herbs Schichimi (page 266)

2 scallions, sliced on the diagonal

Soak the kelp noodles in warm water for 30 minutes, and then rinse. If the noodles are very long, you can cut them with a pair of scissors.

Divide the noodles evenly among four bowls. Top each with broccoli, ginger and a plum. Then bring the water to a boil in a medium saucepan. Turn off the heat and let stand for 3 minutes before adding in the genmaicha. Allow to brew, covered, for 3 to 4 minutes. Strain the tea evenly between the four bowls. Top each bowl with the aminos or tamari, nori, schichimi and scallions.

SERVES 4

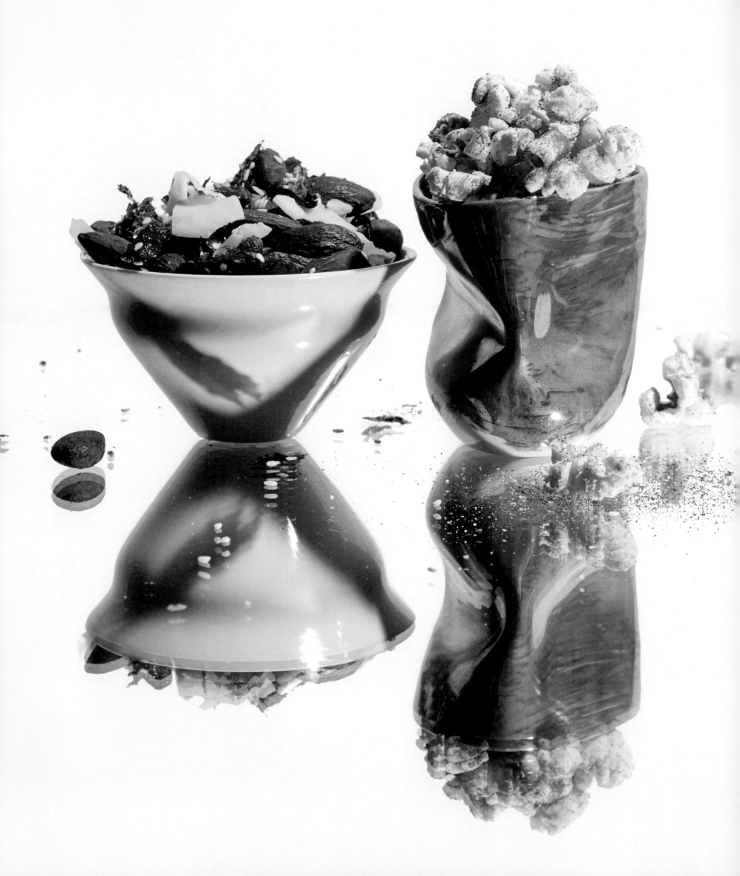

The Japanese seem to do everything right. So, it only stands to reason that we look to their briny-sweet palate for inspiration for this perfect snack mix. Make more than you think you'll need. It's that good. *Arigato,* Kyoto!

KYOTO KRUNCH

1½ cups raw almonds

¼ cup tamari

½ sheet nori

3 tablespoons black or white sesame seeds, toasted

2 tablespoons dulse flakes

1 tablespoon Holy Herbs Schichimi (page 266; optional)

¼ cup dried goji berries

¼ cup dried coconut flakes

Preheat the oven to 300°F. Spread the almonds evenly on a parchment-lined baking sheet and bake for 10 minutes. Transfer to a medium heat-proof bowl and stir in the tamari. Let the almonds absorb the tamari for about 20 minutes, stirring occasionally. Return the soaked almonds to the baking sheet and bake for an additional 20 minutes. When the almonds are done, they will be a bit sticky.

In the meantime, toast the nori by carefully holding it with tongs and waving it over a lit element for 15 to 30 seconds, watching closely. Set aside to cool.

Put the sesame seeds in a dry skillet over medium heat to toast. Watch them closely while shaking the pan, and when they begin to brown, remove from heat.

Add the almonds to a clean medium mixing bowl with the sesame seeds, dulse, and schichimi (if using). Stir well to combine. Set aside until cool. It will continue to crisp.

In the meantime, fold the nori, and, using kitchen shears, cut it into thin strips (approximately 1 inch by ¼ inch).

Add the nori, berries and coconut. Stir well to combine.

MAKES 2½ CUPS

This light, brighter take on traditional hummus embodies spring. The perfect dinner prep snack, it pairs well with crudité, raw crackers and a glass of something cold.

BEGIN AGAIN HUMMUS

2 cups fresh shell peas

¼ cup tahini

Juice of ½ lemon

½ teaspoon
Himalayan pink salt

¼ cup mint leaves

Add all ingredients to a food processor and blend to combine. Taste and adjust seasonings, if desired.

MAKES 2½ CUPS

A throwback to 1970s cocktail fare, these boatlike canapés are reborn for High Vibrational times. Come sail away.

GREEN GODDESSES

1 cup Sunflower
Ricotta (page 253)

½ cup chopped fresh
herbs (chives, parsley,
basil, tarragon, mint
and/or cilantro)

¼ teaspoon salt, plus
more for sprinkling

Squeeze of lemon juice

Leaves from
1 to 2 heads endive
or romaine hearts

Olive oil, to taste

Combine the ricotta, herbs, salt and lemon juice in a small mixing bowl. Stuff each lettuce leaf with the ricotta mixture. Drizzle the "boats" with oil and a sprinkle of salt.

SERVES MANY

Conjuring up the Spanish countryside, this earthy, smoky snack elevates movie night. Almodóvar would approve.

SEVILLA SMOKED POPCORN

3½ tablespoons coconut oil, divided

½ cup popcorn kernels

1 tablespoon smoky paprika

1 teaspoon Himalayan pink salt, plus more if desired

2 tablespoons nutritional yeast, plus more, if desired

Heat a large heavy-bottomed pan (one with a lid) over medium heat. Melt 1½ tablespoons of the oil. Toss a couple of popcorn kernels into the pan and wait for them to pop. This will let you know when the oil is the right temperature. Pour the rest of the kernels into the pan and cover. Once the kernels start popping, shake the pan every 10 seconds or so until the popping starts to slow down. Remove the pan from the heat and continue to shake for 30 seconds. Transfer half the popcorn to a large bowl.

Mix the remaining 2 tablespoons of coconut oil, the paprika, salt and yeast in a small saucepan. Whisk over low heat until the oil is melted and the ingredients are blended. Remove from the heat and pour half into the bowl with the popcorn. Toss to combine. Add the remaining popcorn and the remaining spice mixture to the bowl and toss again. Adjust seasonings, to taste.

SERVES 2

NOTE: Feel free to pop the popcorn any way you like. We love a Whirly Pop!

So nice, you'll make it twice. And, with an extra one on hand, you won't need to hoard it. This tart dessert makes the perfect breakfast, so be sure you have enough for the morning after. And, the morning after that. Wake up to the bright and shining flavors of spring.

SPRING-AWAKENING CRUMBLE

1 cup gluten-free oats, divided

½ cup coconut flour

½ cup sunflower seeds

1 teaspoon cinnamon

½ cup maple syrup

1 tablespoon coconut oil

½ teaspoon Himalayan pink salt

3 cups chopped strawberries

½ cup goji berries

½ teaspoon vanilla extract or ¼ vanilla bean

Juice of 1 lemon

1 tablespoon coconut sugar

1 tablespoon arrowroot

Om Chantilly (page 264)

Preheat the oven to 350°F.

Place ½ cup of the oats in a high-speed blender, and blend until completely broken down. Transfer to a large mixing bowl and add the remaining ½ cup oats, flour, sunflower seeds, cinnamon, syrup, oil and salt. Mix well, and set aside.

In another medium mixing bowl combine strawberries, goji berries, vanilla, lemon and sugar. Transfer into a medium-size baking dish. Top fruit filling with the oat mixture. Bake for 20 minutes, then rotate and bake for another 15 to 20 minutes, or until the top becomes golden brown and the filling starts to bubble up. Serve with Om Chantilly.

SERVES 6

Anglophiles, rejoice! Our take on the classic Eton mess is here. Filled with farm fresh strawberries, coconut cream and a magical meringue made only from plants, this version is top notch. And easy peasy.

STRAWBERRY FOOL

1 pint strawberries, stemmed and chopped coarsely

2 tablespoons coconut sugar

1 tablespoon apple cider vinegar or balsamic vinegar

Om Chantilly (page 264)

Toasted coconut flakes

Place half the strawberries, sugar and vinegar in a medium mixing bowl and massage well. Allow to sit for 10 minutes. Then, transfer the macerated strawberries to a high-speed blender and puree. Fold the puree into the whipped cream. Whip the cream, if necessary, then fold in the remaining strawberries. Top with the coconut flakes and a few more strawberries, if desired.

SERVES 4

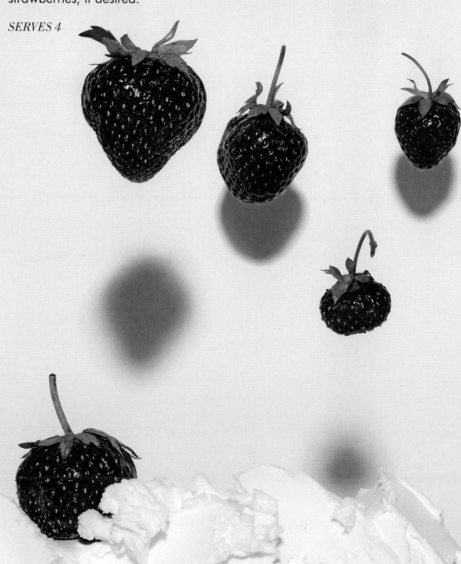

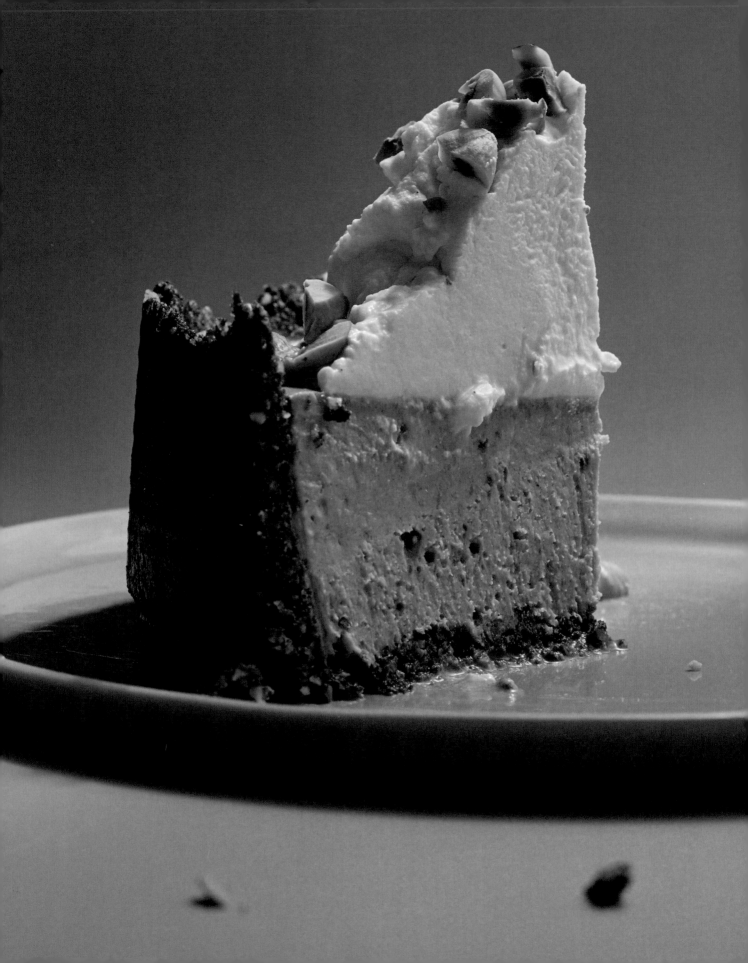

A perfect pie for the disbeliever. This rich, decadent dessert hits all the right notes. Loaded with superfoods, healthy fats, and nostalgia, it's loved by kids and adults alike. The crust is laced with reishi, supporting yin energy and offering immune support, and the filling is spiked with tocotrienols and pine pollen, encouraging glowing skin and creativity, while the lemon adds a surprising brightness. This is pie reinvented.

THE QUEEN HEALER CREAM PIE

1½ cups walnuts, soaked overnight*

1 cup raw cacao powder, plus more for garnish

2 teaspoons reishi

4 to 6 large fresh medjool dates, pitted

FILLING
1½ cups cashews

½ cup coconut oil, melted

5 medjool dates, pitted

¼ cup fresh lemon juice

3 bananas

¼ cup tocotrienols

1 cup coconut milk

2 teaspoons vanilla extract

½ teaspoon Himalayan pink salt

2 tablespoons pine pollen, plus more for garnish

WHIPPED CREAM
1 can coconut cream, chilled

½ teaspoon vanilla extract (optional)

½ cup filberts, soaked overnight* and chopped

Place the walnuts, cacao and reishi in the bowl of a food processor and pulse until crumbly. Add 4 roughly chopped dates and continue pulsing until sticky. You may need to add more dates. Press the mixture into a 9-inch springform pan, covering the bottom and about 1 to 2 inches up the sides. Set aside.

To make the filling: Place all the ingredients in a powerful blender and blend until smooth. Pour over the nut crust and chill overnight, or until set.

Add the coconut cream and vanilla (if using) into a large cool mixing bowl. With an electric mixer, beat until whipped and light. Top the pie with the whipped cream, and garnish with a sprinkling of pine pollen, chopped filberts and cacao.

SERVES 10 OR MAKES ONE 9-INCH PIE

Soaking the nuts removes hard-to-digest phytic acid, but if time does not allow, this pie will still work well.

REISHI

Known in some circles as the queen healer, reishi is an adaptogenic mushroom revered by both Eastern and Western healers. Generally taken as a tea or tonic herb, reishi is said to support immune function, encourage healthy sleep and combat anxiety and stress. But traditional Chinese medicine also recognizes reishi for its spiritual side. In this light, reishi is a shen tonic, supporting our fertile and creative energies and bringing lightness and inward awareness to the body. You can find reishi in supplement form, but we like reishi powder to add into our tonic drinks and even our raw chocolates and desserts. There are many varieties of reishi, from red to purple to the very rare white, so look for a supplement that delivers a blend. Balance the body, awaken the spirit. Hail to the queen.

We adapted this recipe from one of our favorite healthy bloggers, McKel Hill of Nutrition Stripped. Of course, we love that the base is made with coconut butter, which becomes a perfect vehicle for our favorite flavors. This variation takes us to Japan and back. We call these dessert, but, more often than not, we eat one (or a few!) for breakfast.

LIFE FORCE BONBONS

1 (16-ounce) jar of coconut butter

⅓ cup coconut oil

1 tablespoon maple syrup

Pinch of Himalayan sea salt

2 tablespoons matcha

1 teaspoon ground cardamom

Add the coconut butter, oil, syrup and salt to a medium heatproof bowl. Set the bowl over a saucepan of shallow simmering water on low heat to create a double boiler. Stir until melted and combined. Turn off the heat and stir in the matcha and cardamom.

Pour into standard-size chocolate molds and chill. Store refrigerated in an airtight container.

MAKES 16 1.25-OUNCE BONBONS

NOTES: We like silicone molds, but for other materials, you may want to lightly grease them with some coconut oil.

If you don't have chocolate molds, pour a thin layer into a parchment-lined jelly roll pan and cut once chilled. As your first round chills, the mixture can sit on the stovetop. You may need to gently rewarm it to create a liquid consistency before pouring again.

Crispy chocolate shell done right, this High Vibe "nice cream" takes us back to childhood. Soft serve just got a whole lot better!

STRAWBERRY NICE CREAM WITH SPICY CHOCOLATE CRISPY SHELL

5 or 6 strawberries

1 tablespoon tocotrienols

Splash of nut milk

Splash of vanilla extract

Pinch of Himalayan pink salt

3 or 4 ripe bananas, frozen and cut into pieces

CRISPY SHELL

⅛ cup raw cacao powder

⅛ cup Hot Hot Chocolate (page 248)

¼ cup coconut oil, melted

2 teaspoons honey

Splash of vanilla extract

Pinch of Himalayan pink salt

Add the strawberries, tocotrienols, nut milk, vanilla and salt into a blender or food processor and blend until combined. Add the bananas, and blend until it's the consistency of soft serve ice cream. Scoop into chilled bowls, or place it in the freezer for a more traditional ice cream texture.

For the crispy shell: place all ingredients in a bowl, blender or food processor. Whisk or blend until combined and the consistency is like chocolate syrup. Pour over Nice Cream, and watch the magic happen.

SERVES 2 TO 4

TOCOTRIENOLS

This airy and sweet vanilla powder is actually a rice-bran soluble, or the bran of the rice minus the fiber. Tocotrienols are packed with vitamins D and E, making them a genuine beauty food. We use tocotrienols much like a high vibe nondairy creamer, adding them to our teas and tonic drinks to deliver a mellow, creamy sweetness. Add to smoothies, or eat by the spoonful straight from the package. Tocotrienols can also be used topically, and our estheticians at CAP Beauty regularly mix them into custom face masks to deliver hydration and a topical hit of vitamin D and vitamin E. There was a time when tocotrienols were impossibly expensive, but sound-wave technology has made them easier to produce. Now, we can spread the love far and wide. Tocotrienols for all!

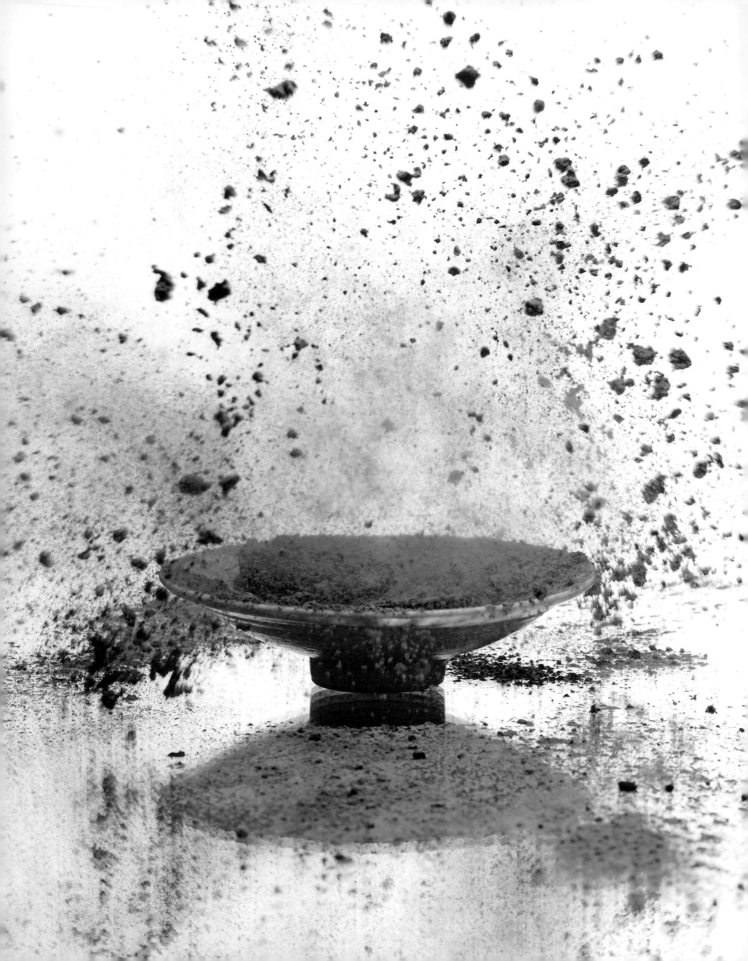

Matcha makes its way into our life on the daily. Whether that's straight up in the morning, a mask in the evening, or these shortbread cookies in the afternoon. Reach for these simple, not so sweet coins, and pair them with your 4 o'clock cup. Afternoons just got better.

ARIGATO! MATCHA COINS

½ teaspoon ground flaxseeds

1 teaspoon hot filtered water

¾ cup gluten-free oats

½ cup pumpkin seeds

¼ teaspoon Himalayan pink salt

2 tablespoons matcha powder

⅓ cup + 1 tablespoon coconut oil

¼ cup coconut sugar

½ teaspoon vanilla extract

In a small bowl, combine the flaxseeds and hot water, and allow to stand for 10 minutes until they reach a gel-like consistency. Set aside.

Place the oats and pumpkin seeds into a high-speed blender and process until finely ground. Transfer into a medium mixing bowl, add the salt and matcha and mix well. Set aside.

In the bowl of a mixer, add the oil and sugar. Beat them on high speed until the sugar has broken down slightly. Then, beat in the vanilla and flax mixture until combined. Transfer half of the oat and pumpkin seed mixture to the mixer and beat until incorporated. Repeat with the other half. Remove the batter onto a large sheet of parchment paper, and gently press down. Place another parchment paper on top of the dough and roll it out to ¼ to ⅛ inch thick with a rolling pin. Place the parchment paper onto a baking sheet and pop into the refrigerator to chill for about 30 minutes.

Preheat the oven to 325°F. Take off the top layer of parchment and transfer the dough (and the bottom layer of parchment) to a flat surface. Make coin shapes in the dough by using a round cookie cutter. Transfer the cookies to a parchment-lined baking sheet (you can reuse the top layer of parchment from before). Bake for 10 to 12 minutes. Remove and allow to cool.

MAKES 15 TO 25 COINS, DEPENDING ON THE SIZE OF THE CUTTER

Warm yourself from the inside out. This modernized take on a classic dessert relies on the power of thermogenic spices to electrify you from within. Light up, and dig in.

ELECTRIC LIFE TAPIOCA

⅓ cup tapioca pearls

1 cup filtered water

1 can full-fat coconut milk

2 tablespoons maple syrup

1 teaspoon vanilla extract or ½ vanilla bean

2 apricots, chopped, plus more for garnish

1 tablespoon chia seeds

1 teaspoon ground dandelion root

1 teaspoon cinnamon

½ teaspoon ginger

⅛ teaspoon cayenne

⅛ teaspoon ground black pepper

½ teaspoon Himalayan pink salt

Coconut flakes, toasted

In a small bowl, soak the tapioca in the water for at least 30 minutes. Transfer to a medium saucepan and add the coconut milk, syrup, vanilla, apricots, chia seeds, dandelion, cinnamon, ginger, cayenne, black pepper and salt. Heat over medium-low heat until boiling. Reduce heat to a simmer and cook until most of the liquid has been absorbed, stirring often. Remove from the heat, and allow the pudding to cool, then transfer to the refrigerator to chill. Top with coconut flakes and chopped apricots and serve.

MAKES 4 CUPS/4 TO 6 SERVINGS

Matcha is a religion at CAP Beauty. This bright and earthy Japanese green tea powder encourages calm, focus and a clean, steady energy. It's no wonder that the masters of meditation have used matcha for centuries. Our day isn't complete without our matcha rituals, whether we drink it neat or create this delicious High Vibe latte. Join the cult.

MASTERMIND LATTE

6 ounces nut milk

½ teaspoon matcha

1 teaspoon coconut butter

1 tablespoon of tocotrienols

In a small saucepan over low heat, gently warm the nut milk. Whisk in the matcha and continue to warm, stirring continuously. Be careful not to bring to a boil. Add the coconut butter and tocotrienols, and whisk vigorously until blended. Pour into your favorite tea bowl or mug and enjoy. *Oishii!*

SERVES 1

Another nod to the islands, this bright-and-light juice is simply divine. Perfect on its own or served over ice with sparkling mineral water. Afternoon bubbly, CAP Beauty style.

THE ISLANDS

½ pineapple

2 cucumbers

Handful of mint

Sparkling mineral water (optional)

Juice the pineapple, cucumbers and mint in a juicer. Excellent served on its own, or pour over ice and add sparkling mineral water (if using).

SERVES 2

The love child of rhubarb and kombucha, a probiotic heavy, fermented brew, this tart and refreshing drink takes advantage of spring's bounty. Nutrient dense and delicious, this cooler is one to be savored. Feel the love, and drink it in. We like to look for locally made kombuchas, but also go for larger brands like GT's. If you can find them, Health-Ade and Pilot are great local brands.

THE SPRING HAS SPRUNG KOMBUCHA FRAPPE

4 cups rhubarb, chopped

1 tablespoon fresh lemon juice

1 teaspoon ground coriander

1 tablespoon coconut sugar

1 (16-ounce) bottle unflavored kombucha

1 cup ice cubes

Preheat the oven to 400°F. In a large baking dish, combine the rhubarb, lemon juice, coriander and sugar, and mix together well. Cover and bake for 20 minutes. Uncover and bake for an additional 10 minutes. Allow to cool and then transfer to a high-speed blender and blend until combined. Add the ice cubes and kombucha and blend once more, tamping down, if necessary. Divide between glasses and serve immediately.

SERVES 4

Sea buckthorn berries are a favorite ingredient at CAP Beauty for their hydrating and healing powers. Grown at high altitudes, they're a leading source of omega-7s, the beauty omega, known for strengthening hair, encouraging luminous skin and stronger nails. We've grown to love their bracing tart taste. Paired with bitters, the superhero of gut and digestive health, this is an immune-supportive, beauty-boosting tonic. Pucker up, and drink it in.

SEA BUCKTHORN SPRITZER

2 tablespoons pureed sea buckthorn berries*

Splash of bitters

6 ounces sparking mineral water

Place the sea buckthorn and bitters in your favorite glass. Gently stir and pour sparkling water on top.

SERVES 1

*You can buy sea buckthorn berry puree at capbeauty.com, or through other online retailers.

Perfectly pink, this nectar of the Gods is a staple in our fridge. Filled with antioxidants, it's lightly sweet and infuses our milks and teas with Far-East superfood magic.

GOJI NECTAR

1 cup goji berries, soaked overnight

3 cups filtered water

Homemade nut milk (optional)

Add the berries, water and nut milk (if using) to a powerful blender and blend. Enjoy on its own, or add to teas or nut milk.

SERVES MANY

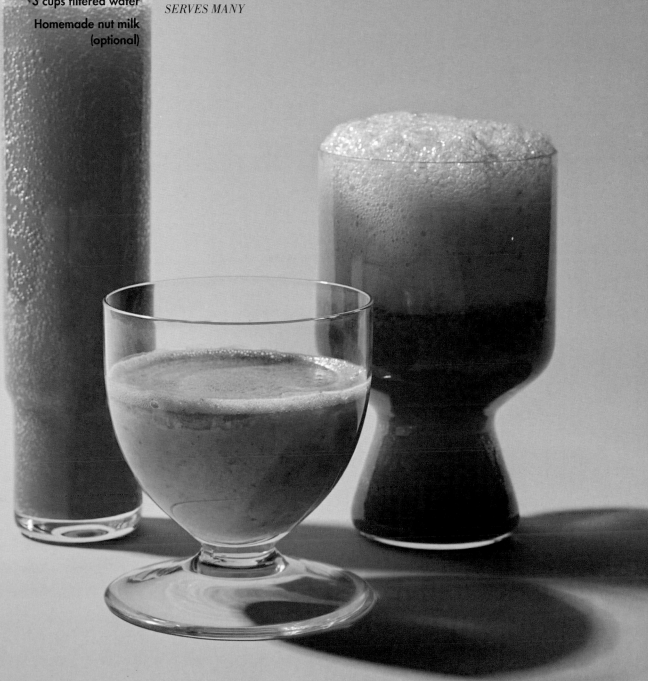

SUMMER

AN INTRO TO SUMMER: HEAVENLY LIGHT

Let there be light. And, let it in. The balmy beautiful days of summer invite spontaneity. Longer days deliver more time for play, for exploring the wonders of nature and for loving, laughing and learning. summer is a siren. Let her sultry ways seduce you. This year, decide for yourself to embrace summer in all her glory. Have a summer fling with summer.

The recipes and rituals shared here showcase summer's glorious bounty. From eating fresh raw foods to kissing the Sun, we raise our vibration by tapping directly into Source. Let the Sun shine in. And on, and on, and on.

SUMMER LOVING

THE SUMMER SKIN PROGRAM

PERFORM: Once or twice daily

WHAT YOU'LL NEED: Cleanser, toner and lighter oils or moisturizers, plus sun protection and a purifying mask

DURATION: 5 to 10 minutes

Keep it light. In hot and humid climates, a little goes a long way. We still encourage a committed skincare routine, but many of us lighten up on the richer products that we use during the rest of the year. Similar to the way our heavier meals give way to salads and juices all summer, our skincare routines become more fresh and clean. An emphasis on cleansing and purifying the skin becomes our main focus, along with healthy sun exposure. We take to tricks like carrying a purifying hydrosol in our bags. Look for one with bacteria-fighting silver to stave off breakouts and congestion. We also love to store products in the fridge for a cooling treat. Try this with hydrosols or moisturizing gels. A probiotic mist is another great addition for keeping unfriendly bacteria at bay and creating a healthy biome on your skin's surface.

We're big believers in absorbing vitamin D on the daily, so we encourage some sun exposure during the healthiest hours, mornings and late afternoons. A sunscreen is imperative, especially at the beach or in other highly reflective settings. It's vital to look for a sunscreen that derives its protection factor by creating a physical barrier, literally blocking the skin's exposure to the sun. When we block the sun's rays, we don't need to rely on chemicals to protect us from the effects of the sun. Look for a sunscreen with zinc oxide as its active ingredient. If you have darker skin, zinc may leave behind a white residue, so you may prefer a tinted version. There are also many ingredients that support sun protection that are not considered sunscreens. Loading up on these antioxidant-rich ingredients can fortify your defenses and prevent further damage. Some of our favorite ingredients to look for are: red raspberry seed oil, carrot seed oil, macadamia nut oil and hemp seed oil. Finally, during the brightest hours, seek shade, invest in a good hat and time your beach trips wisely. There's nothing more beautiful than an early morning or late afternoon at the beach. You'll avoid the crowds and beat the heat.

HOW TO DO IT: Follow the protocol from spring (see page 10), swapping heavier oils and creams for lighter versions. In every season, but especially in summer, add a zinc oxide–based sunscreen as a final step in your morning routine. For more-congested and clogged skin, add a purifying mask weekly. Throw on a hat, and get outside.

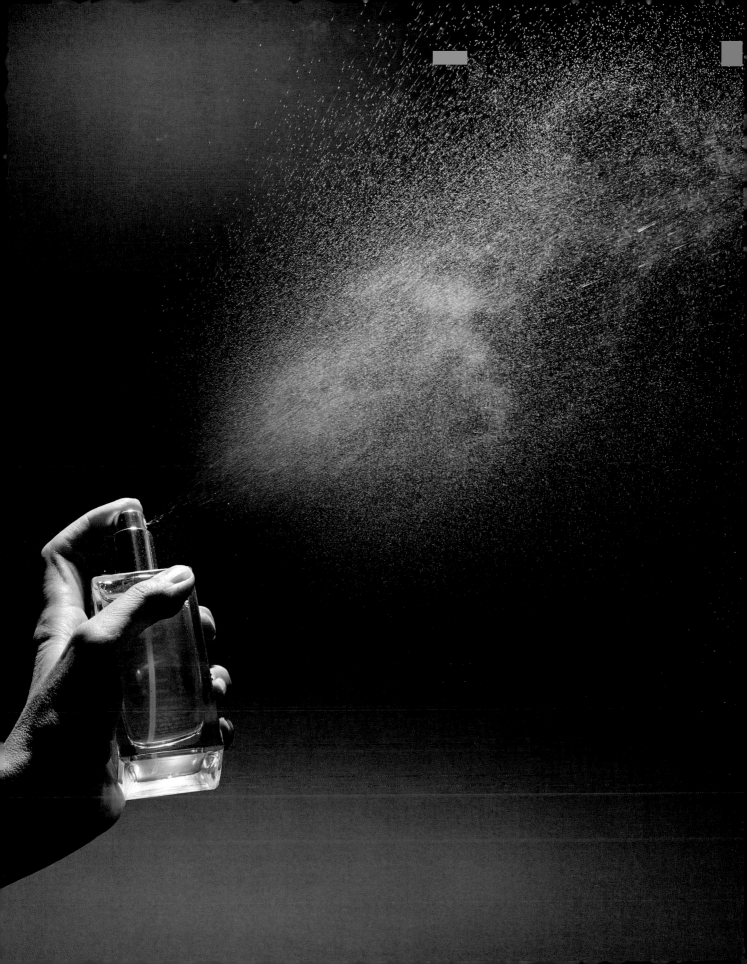

THE SUN WORSHIPPER'S DIET

Eat the rainbow. The antioxidants found in the most vibrant fruits and vegetables fortify your skin from the inside out. We've said it before: Begin within. By adding in these superior foods, we help our skin create a stronger defense against sun damage. A sunburn is essentially inflammation of your largest organ, and so, by eating an abundance of anti-inflammatory foods, we help to heal this state. And, just as important, avoid foods that cause inflammation. So, steer clear of the fry shack, and hit the mango hut instead. Color is your clue. Get your hands on as many fruits and vegetables as possible, the more colorful, the better. Be the rainbow.

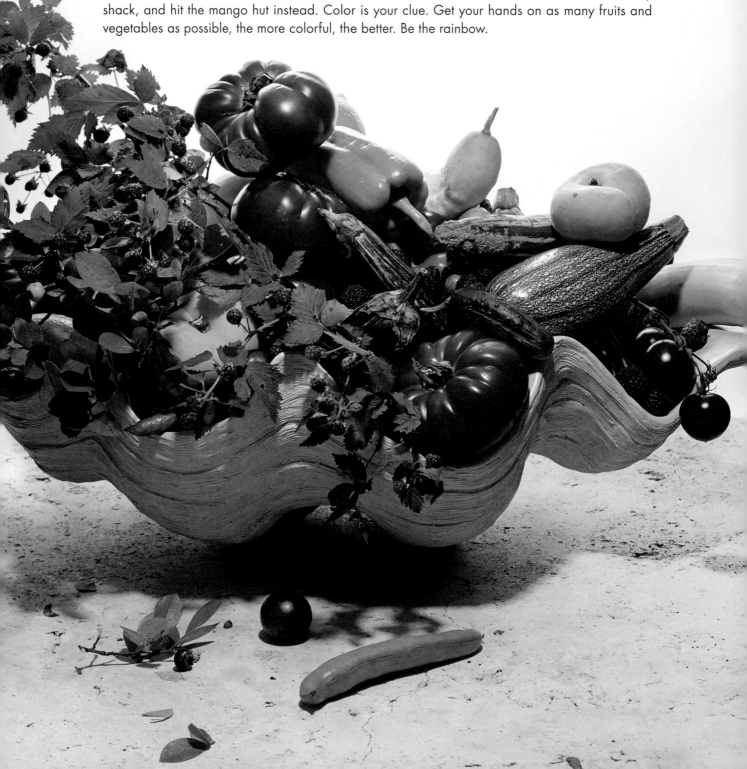

PEDI-CARE

Put your best foot forward. Literally. summer can leave your feet exposed and wanting for some love. Take a few minutes to take care of your over-worked feet. One of our favorite activities at the end of a long, hot day is a quick-and-cooling scrub and soak in a basin or tub. This post-work ritual cools you down and maintains pretty feet for the sandal season at hand. Don't overcomplicate this. A quick wash and some daily love goes a long way. Your feet will thank you.

HOW TO DO IT: Wash your feet under vigorously running cool water. We like to sit on the edge of the tub for this. Using your scrub or pumice, exfoliate your feet, focusing on the most calloused areas. You can also use a small brush to clean the toenails. Rinse well, dry off and moisturize. Throw on socks or slippers.

PERFORM:
Once daily

WHAT YOU'LL NEED:
A tub or deep sink, a scrub or pumice stone, an optional nail brush, moisturizer and socks or slippers

DURATION:
3 to 5 minutes

SUMMER COOLING MASK

Our CAP Beauty family has become obsessed with the power of a full-fat yogurt mask. One of our brand leaders, Marie Veronique, introduced us to the magic of the lactic acid and beneficial bacteria contained in high quality, live yogurt when used directly on the skin. Acting as a gentle-yet-effective exfoliant, this kitchen staple is a cooling and hydrating treatment for summer skin.

HOW TO DO IT: Spoon ¼ cup plain yogurt into a mixing bowl. Apply the yogurt with a brush to your clean skin and allow it to sit on your skin for 5 to 10 minutes. Rinse thoroughly, and apply your favorite oil or serum to your freshly revealed skin.

PERFORM: Once or twice a week

WHAT YOU'LL NEED: Full-fat plain yogurt with live and active cultures, a small mixing bowl and a brush

DURATION:
5 to 10 minutes

SUMMER PRODUCT RECOMMENDATIONS

CLEANSER: Dr. Alkaitis Organic Purifying Facial Cleanser, Tata Harper Purifying Cleanser, EiR Active Face Wash

HYDROSOL: Linné Refresh Face Mist, Odacité Rose + Neroli Treatment Mist, May Lindstrom The Jasmine Garden

MOISTURIZER: Shiva Rose Glow Face Balm, Keys Solar Rx Moisturizer, Pai Avocado and Jojoba Hydrating Day Cream

SUN PROTECTION: Kypris Pot of Shade, Raw Elements Eco Tint Stick 30, de Mamiel Exhale Daily Hydrating Nectar

OTHER GOOD STUFF: In Fiore Soleil Fleur, Hannes Dottir Seamasque, Wildcare Soft Focus Coconut Milk Mask

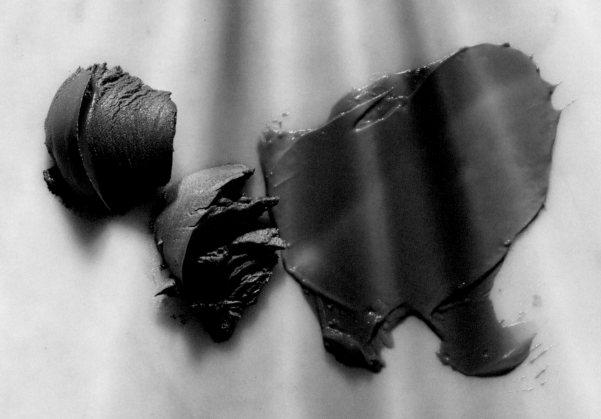

THE SUMMER MAKEUP PALETTE

Long days and warm nights inspire our summer colors. Look to the sunset to highlight sun-kissed skin. Corals, peaches, pinks and gold fade into bright white and dramatic black. Abandon old ways of thinking about color, and let your inner siren guide you. Get creative with your palette, and feel the heat. Let these hues reflect your perfect summer day and sultry warm night. Let this be your summer of love.

BE A SPORT

Shake up your routine, and make exercise a game. Skip the gym or fitness class and head to the court, the field or the pool. Childhood summers spent playing tag, Marco Polo in the pool and soccer with friends kept us active (and tan and fit!) until the sun went down. Channel your inner child, and find delight in sport and movement. Next time you're at the beach, join a pickup volleyball game, take a surf lesson or fly a kite. The idea is to get moving, and have a ball.

SCRUB IT OUT

Get scrubbing and reveal smooth and energized skin. By removing top, often dead, layers of skin, we uncover the soft and youthful skin that lives below. Summer's environmental stressors can create a dense and protective layer that feels and looks rough. And, products have a harder time penetrating hardened skin, so by removing this layer, we let in the nutrition and conditioning that products deliver. Take it off, and find your softer side.

HOW TO DO IT: You can mix up your own natural scrub by mixing ½ cup coconut, olive or other oil with ½ cup salt, sugar and/or coffee grounds. Get undressed and step into the tub. Starting at your feet, apply the scrub and rub in circular motions, working your way up your body, stopping at your neck. Take your time, and go for as long as you like. Fifteen to 20 minutes is ideal, though that can feel like an eternity. Put on your favorite podcast or playlist, and tune in to tune out.

The scrub will most likely land all over the tub, making it slippery, so be careful. Don't forget to wash the tub out afterward, as there will be residue from the oil. When you're ready, shower to remove the scrub and feel the soft and hydrated skin beneath. Don your favorite sundress, and enjoy your new beauty.

PERFORM: Once or twice a week

WHAT YOU'LL NEED: Body scrub

DURATION: As long as you can, plus time for a shower

THE DIET OF DISCOVERY

PERFORM:
Once, or as needed

WHAT YOU'LL NEED:
A journal

DURATION:
1 to 2 months

Know thyself. We've stressed the importance of self-discovery, of tuning in to reveal what makes you thrive and what, on the contrary, may hinder your flight. An elimination diet is a controlled experiment designed to shed light on the foods that cause your body distress. There are blood tests for this, but these can be costly and may not always reveal the more subtle culprits. An elimination diet is free and connects you to your body in a deeper way. We recommend this to everyone, even those already eating a very clean diet. And, because of the abundance of fresh fruits and vegetables, summer is the ideal time to dive in.

HOW TO DO IT: For 3 weeks, eliminate from your diet the most common allergens: gluten, dairy, eggs and soy. In addition, avoid any other foods that you suspect may be trouble for you and cause you discomfort after eating. These may even include some healthy foods. Remember that the point of this is to discover what works best for you and your body. Nuts and seeds, grains, yeast, citrus fruit, beans and most sugars are other likely stressors, as are most nightshades. These include white potatoes, tomatoes, eggplant, peppers, goji berries and tomatillos. Be honest with yourself, and cut out the likely offenders. We also recommend avoiding alcohol during this time. It's important to really connect to how you feel and a hangover, even a subtle one, clouds this connection. Finally, remember that processed foods often contain hidden ingredients, so steer clear of those, too.

The next 3 weeks will take some discipline, but you'll feel great, and the knowledge you gain from this experiment may revolutionize the way you feel. Tune in and keep a journal, noting any changes to the conditions that plague you, from acne to fatigue to brain fog, digestive stress, achy joints and sleeplessness. Are you feeling good? We bet you are. Stick with it.

At the end of this 21-day period, pick one food category to reintroduce. Note any symptoms or changes to how you feel. How is your digestion? Your ability to focus? Any changes to your skin? Or to the level of heat you feel in your body? Obviously, if you notice any symptoms, eliminate this food group from your diet and embrace the shift. After 3 days, you can reintroduce another category. Keep adding foods back in, noting any that don't agree with you.

Remember, it's vital to add just one category at a time so you can truly isolate any culprits. If you break the elimination period with a slice of pizza and then suffer a spell of breakouts, you won't know if it's the gluten, the dairy or even the tomatoes that trigger you. Be controlled. A friend of ours thought she was allergic to gluten, until a strict elimination diet revealed that it was actually yeast that caused her migraines, knowledge that has changed her life.

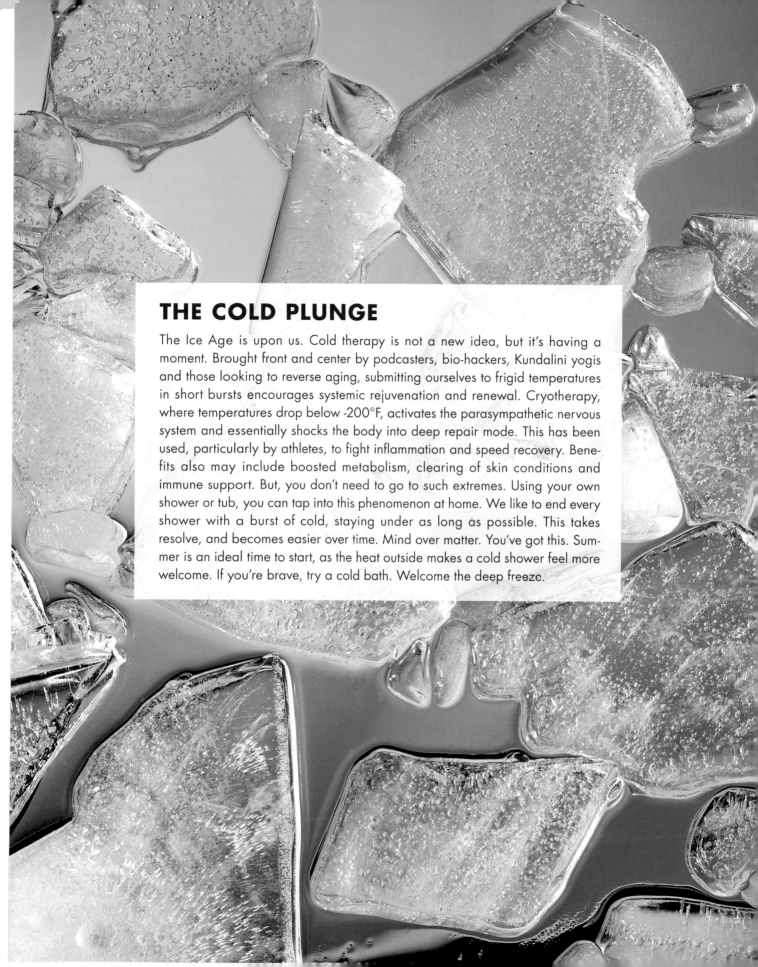

THE COLD PLUNGE

The Ice Age is upon us. Cold therapy is not a new idea, but it's having a moment. Brought front and center by podcasters, bio-hackers, Kundalini yogis and those looking to reverse aging, submitting ourselves to frigid temperatures in short bursts encourages systemic rejuvenation and renewal. Cryotherapy, where temperatures drop below -200°F, activates the parasympathetic nervous system and essentially shocks the body into deep repair mode. This has been used, particularly by athletes, to fight inflammation and speed recovery. Benefits also may include boosted metabolism, clearing of skin conditions and immune support. But, you don't need to go to such extremes. Using your own shower or tub, you can tap into this phenomenon at home. We like to end every shower with a burst of cold, staying under as long as possible. This takes resolve, and becomes easier over time. Mind over matter. You've got this. Summer is an ideal time to start, as the heat outside makes a cold shower feel more welcome. If you're brave, try a cold bath. Welcome the deep freeze.

HEART-OPENING CRYSTALS

These are the stones we keep on hand to let in the light and open the heart. Float through summer, and stay high.

ROSE QUARTZ: This may be the official crystal of CAP Beauty. When we built our West Village store, we embedded this pink stone under the floors and in our foundation. We wanted CAP Beauty to radiate love, so we turned to this heart opening and love producing crystal. Let it be your official stone of summer.

RHODONITE: This new wave beauty vibrates love and encourages a state of calm.

RHODOCHROSITE: Be awash in love with this creativity-inducing stone.

PERIDOT: This highly spiritual stone calls forth love and beauty, but only for those ready to engage on a higher plane.

GREEN JASPER: This calming stone strengthens resolve and builds fortitude. Dispel negativity and ensure sound rest.

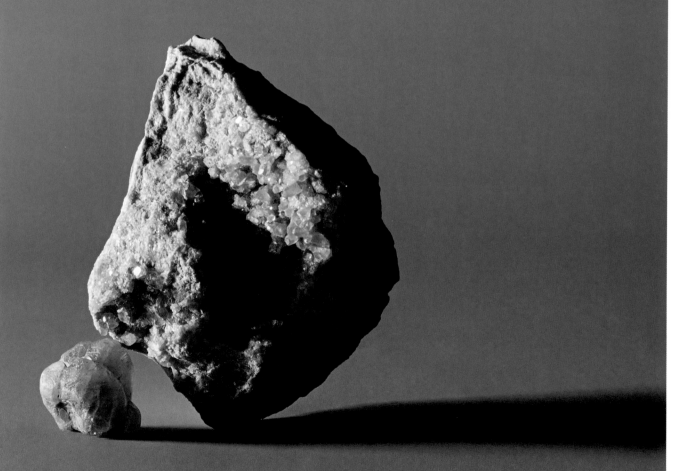

FLOWER POWER

Our love for Japan runs deep. Especially when it comes to flowers. *Ikebana*, the Japanese art of flower arrangement, derives its beauty from the philosophy of merging indoors and outdoors, man with nature. In *Ikebana*, cuttings of branches, blossoms, twigs and grasses are brought indoors and arranged in a single vessel. And, while diverse in materials, each arrangement is simple and practical. Use what grows in the yard or what you forage from your local park (no cutting). Pick up fallen branches and sticks. Supplement with a trip to the flower shop, if needed. Keep it considered. You don't need a lot of anything here. The beauty of *Ikebana* lies in its perfect edit, its sparseness and its thoughtful placement. It also happens to be an easy way to add life and vitality to the smaller spaces that some of us in urban areas live in. Let nature in.

PERFORM: Anytime

WHAT YOU'LL NEED:
A beautiful vase, flowers, branches and sticks

DURATION:
30 minutes

SET IT AND FORGET IT

With daytripping and the beach-bound weekends of summer, there's less time to tend to our homes. And, we don't mind. We can spend more time enjoying the sun when we stay on task by utilizing the power of the timer. So often, a simple task begets another and another until we've lost track of what we set out to do in the first place. The ticking timer keeps us honest. A stack of mail waiting to be sorted, a fridge needing to be cleaned or even a fast apartment cleanup is made more effective when we set a time limit and hold ourselves accountable. Twenty minutes to a clean apartment. Whenever Kerrilynn does this and her husband, John, comes home, he can't believe the difference. It's always surprising how a short yet focused bit of time can transform something so radically. You can do it. When the timer is ticking, you won't be led astray. Ticktock.

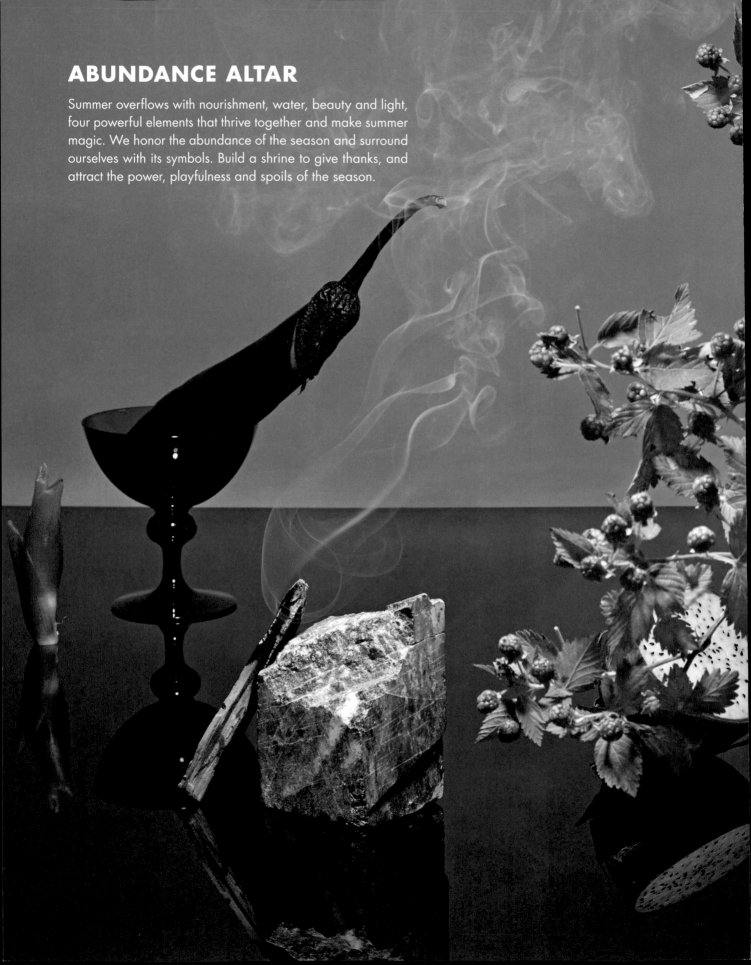

ABUNDANCE ALTAR

Summer overflows with nourishment, water, beauty and light, four powerful elements that thrive together and make summer magic. We honor the abundance of the season and surround ourselves with its symbols. Build a shrine to give thanks, and attract the power, playfulness and spoils of the season.

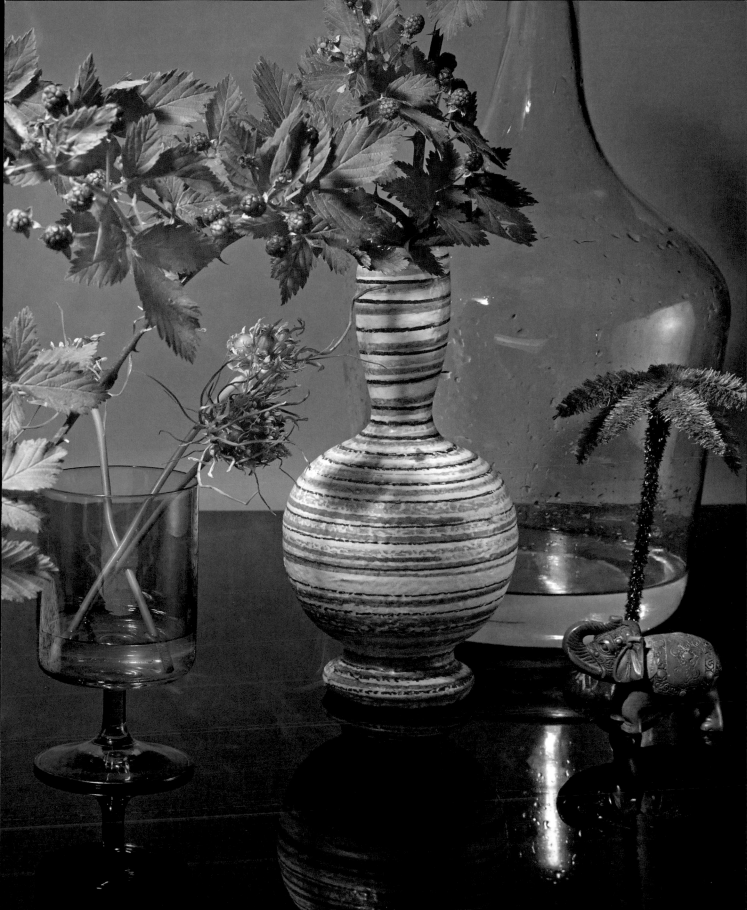

COMPOST THE MOST

PERFORM: Daily,
or when possible
WHAT YOU'LL NEED:
A bowl and
paper bag
DURATION: Seconds

Connect with the cycle of life. One man's trash becomes the riches to fuel new growth. The simple act of setting aside our food scraps for the compost pile allows us all to be farmers for a day. If you aren't a gardener and don't keep a compost pile in your yard, you can still put your scraps to good use. Many cities now include composting programs and even pick up curbside. Others can find community compost drop-offs at their local farmer's markets. We contribute to our soil health and reduce waste through this simple ritual. Feed your food.

HOW TO DO IT: While cooking, set aside any fruit and vegetable scraps. We keep a bowl counter side to collect them. While cleaning up, toss the contents of the bowl into a paper bag and store it in the freezer until drop-off.

LOVING

PLAY TOGETHER, STAY TOGETHER

A wise man (he was actually a monk!) once told us, "The family that plays together, stays together." He was talking about sports. While this may strike you as simple or even irrelevant, these words have stuck with us. Find time to move with your loved ones. There's something in the act of engaging mind and body together that brings us closer and strengthens our bonds. Self care is love, after all. Cindy loves a game of tennis with Laurent and actually took up running to share this with him. Kerrilynn and John hit the yoga mat together every weekend. Get going to gain strength and flexibility in body, mind and relationships!

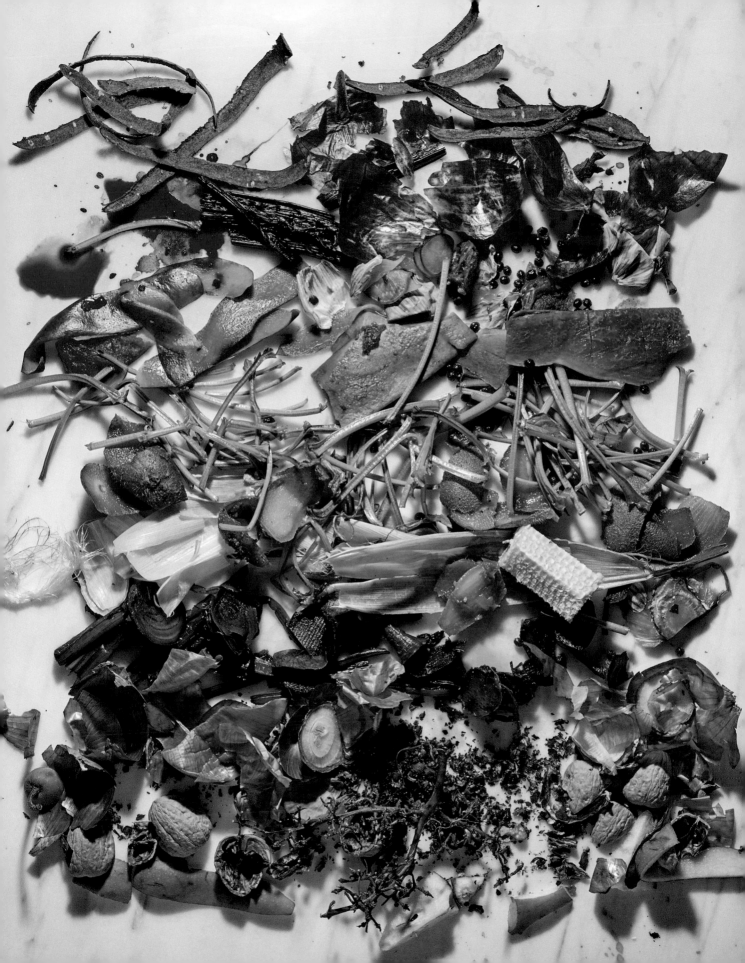

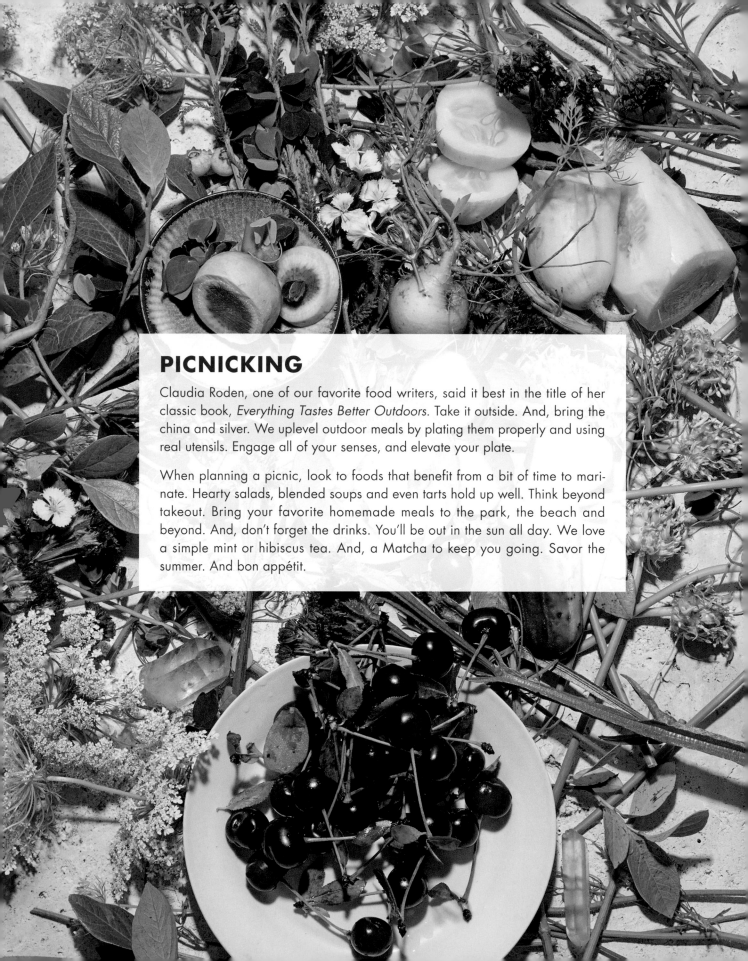

PICNICKING

Claudia Roden, one of our favorite food writers, said it best in the title of her classic book, *Everything Tastes Better Outdoors*. Take it outside. And, bring the china and silver. We uplevel outdoor meals by plating them properly and using real utensils. Engage all of your senses, and elevate your plate.

When planning a picnic, look to foods that benefit from a bit of time to marinate. Hearty salads, blended soups and even tarts hold up well. Think beyond takeout. Bring your favorite homemade meals to the park, the beach and beyond. And, don't forget the drinks. You'll be out in the sun all day. We love a simple mint or hibiscus tea. And, a Matcha to keep you going. Savor the summer. And bon appétit.

A DAY IN THE LIFE:
ECSTATIC SUMMER

GOOD MORNING, SUNSHINE. GREET THE DAY, AND LET THE WARMTH of summer fill your heart. Freedom abounds, and opportunity calls. Stretch it out, and salute the sun, our guiding force. Say your thanks, and tell the universe what you wish for. The possibilities are infinite, and summer is the time for taking. Make your way to the kitchen for a big glass of filtered water with lemon. Spike it with chlorella to up the ante. Alkalize. Don't forget your probiotics. Your body will thank you. Make a morning tonic, and take it hot or cold. We love a cold and frothy summer brew. Then, get outside, and soak it in. A morning workout in the park jump starts the day. Or, better still, meet a friend for tennis. Love, all. Match point. Then, recharge with a cold pressed juice. Make it green, and drink it in. Let the living vibrations course through you. Energize. Get high. Hit the shower. Dry brush first. Scrub it out, and reveal your most beautiful skin. Then, brace yourself for the big chill. End your shower with a blast of cold. Be strong, stick with it and know that your body will benefit from the challenge. A little goes a long way. What does the day hold in store? A trip to the beach? A day at the office? Either way, pack your lunch. A big, fresh salad, nori wraps or a jarful of gazpacho will infuse your system with nutrients and life force. Go for lots of color here. You are the rainbow. Light is on your side. Use the extra time to absorb the good vibrations of summer. A concert in the park or dinner al fresco is calling. Bring your friends, bring your lover, bring your four-legged friends. Bring a Stone Fruit Crumble (see page 103) and bring a tonic drink (see "Tonics" on page 246). Share the power of plants, and stand in the light. The sun is setting, time to thank Mother Earth for all she gives. Let the energy of high summer give way to rest with a calming yoga sequence, followed by your evening meditation. Release yourself in Standing Forward Bend, open the hips through Pigeon and greet your hamstrings in Paschimottanasana (that's Seated Forward Bend). Be still. Before bed, treat yourself to a purifying mask or a quick foot bath. Count your blessings, and enter your dreamscape. A kaleidoscope of light. Praise summer.

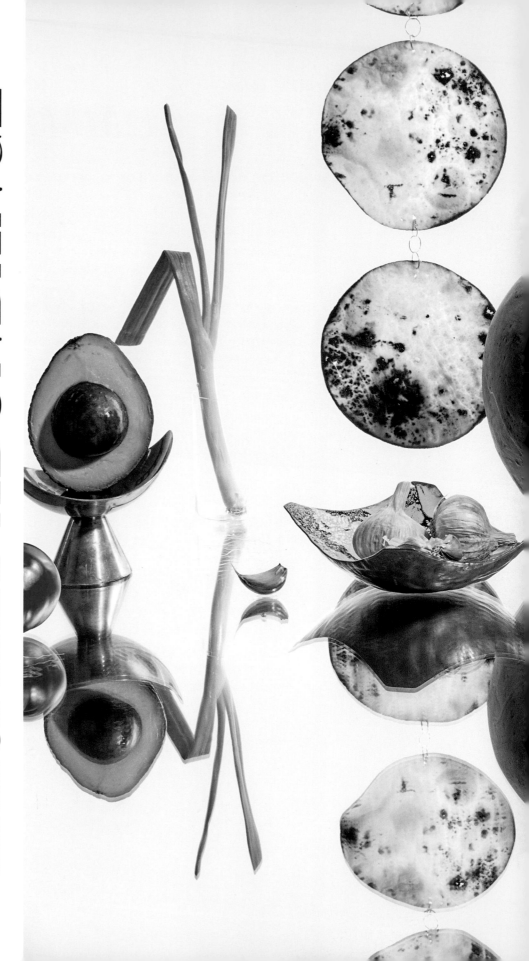

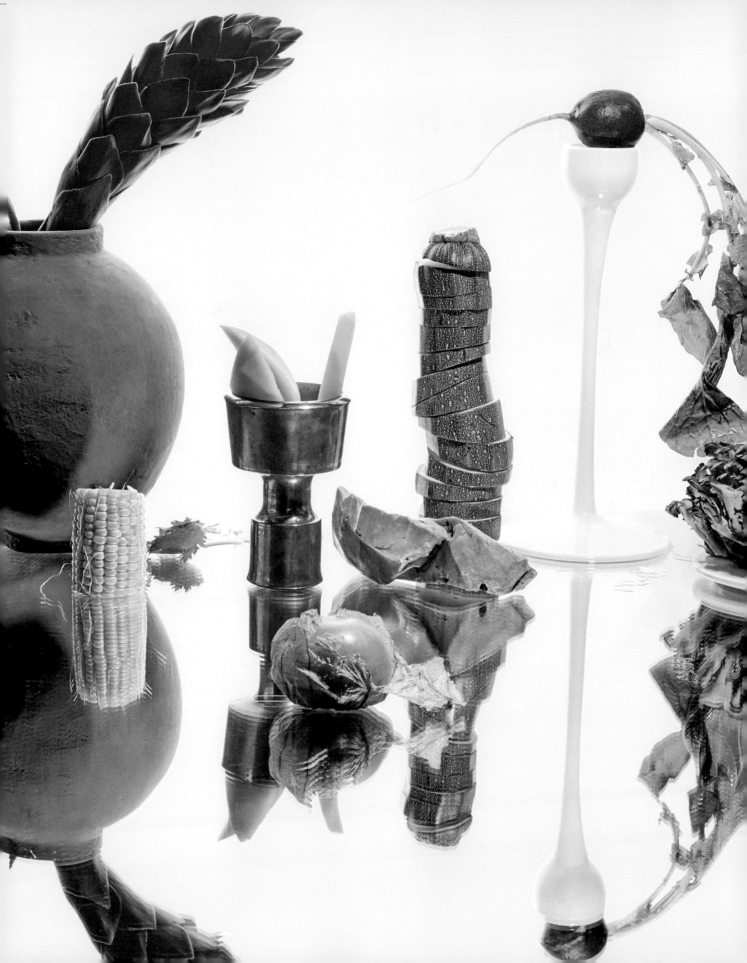

TACO TIME

A taco party is our favorite way to show off the bounty and the power of plants. After all, everyone loves a taco. With endless toppings and unlimited sauces, this south of the border meal pleases all.

Clear the table and make room for the offerings, then let your friends get to work.

HERE'S HOW TO DO IT: Set out all your favorite bowls and fill with any or all of the fillings and toppings below. Set out napkins and plates. Designate a couple of plates for serving freshly warmed tortillas. You may be replenishing these throughout the night, but if you keep them wrapped in a linen napkin, they'll stay warmer longer. Offer fresh romaine leaves as a lighter alternative to tortillas, then let your guests create their own Mexican magic.

Corn tortillas, steamed or heated on the stovetop

Whole romaine leaves, washed and dried

FILLINGS

Roasted Maitake (page 102)

Grilled or roasted zucchini

Perfect Pot of Beans (page 255) made with black beans

TOPPINGS

Cilantro

Radishes

Salsa Verde (page 102)

Pico de Gallo (below)

Minced white onions

Guacamole (opposite)

Pickled jalapeños and carrots (opposite)

Shredded green cabbage

Sauerkraut

Sunflower *Queso* (page 252)

Raw Corn and Mango Salsa (page 102)

Green Goddess Tahini (page 42)

Lime wedges

PICO DE GALLO

1 whole tomato

Big handful of cilantro

½ white onion

½ to 1 jalapeño, seeded (wear plastic gloves when handling)

1 teaspoon apple cider vinegar

Juice of 1 lime

Big pinch of Himalayan pink salt

Add all ingredients to a high-speed blender and blend to the desired consistency.

MAKES 1 CUP

PICKLED JALAPEÑOS AND CARROTS

4 large carrots, sliced thickly on the diagonal

1 white onion, sliced into thick half-rounds

20 jalapeños, seeded and halved (wear plastic gloves when handling)

1½ cups apple cider vinegar

A few big pinches of Himalayan pink salt

1 tablespoon cumin seeds, toasted

1 tablespoon coriander seeds, toasted

Bring a medium pot of water to a boil and prepare an ice water bath. Blanch the carrots. After about 3 minutes, strain and set the carrots in the ice water to stop the cooking. Strain and add to a large glass jar, glass refrigerator dish or nonreactive mixing bowl. Add the onion and jalapeños, and set aside.

Combine the vinegar, salt, cumin, coriander and 1 cup water in a medium saucepan. Bring to a boil over high heat. Turn the heat down to medium and simmer for about 5 minutes. Remove from the heat and carefully pour the vinegar over the vegetables, making sure that the vegetables are completely submerged. Cover the jar or container, and refrigerate for at least 2 days. Store in the refrigerator for up to 3 weeks.

MAKES 1 QUART

GUACAMOLE

3 ripe avocados, pitted

¼ large white onion, finely chopped

Juice of 2 limes, plus more to taste

Big pinch of Himalayan pink salt

Big handful of cilantro, chopped coarsely

Scoop the avocado flesh into a medium bowl. Add the onion, lime juice and salt. Smash the avocados with a large dinner fork and fold together until well mixed. We like a chunky texture but feel free to keep going if you like a smoother mash. Add the cilantro, and mix to distribute evenly. Taste and adjust seasonings, adding more lime juice, if needed. Transfer to a serving bowl and enjoy!

MAKES 1½ CUPS

SALSA VERDE

10 tomatillos, papery shells removed

Big handful of cilantro

½ white onion

½ to 1 jalapeño

Juice of 1 lime

Big pinch of Himalayan pink salt

Over medium high heat, in a dry skillet, roast the tomatillos until slightly charred and softened. Add them and all the remaining ingredients to a high-speed blender and blend to the desired consistency.

MAKES 2 CUPS

RAW CORN AND MANGO SALSA

3 cups fresh corn, cut from cob

1 small jalapeño, seeded and minced (wear plastic gloves when handling)

1 clove garlic, minced

1 mango, chopped

¼ cup coconut mayonnaise

Juice of 1 lime

¼ teaspoon turmeric

½ teaspoon pimenton

¼ teaspoon Himalayan pink salt

½ cup cilantro, chopped

Cracked black pepper

In a large mixing bowl, combine the corn, jalapeño, garlic and mango. Set aside. In a smaller mixing bowl, combine the coconut mayonnaise, lime, turmeric, pimenton and salt. Whisk well to combine. Transfer it along with the cilantro into the bowl with the corn. Crack some black pepper on top, and serve.

MAKES 4 CUPS

MAITAKE

Another magical mushroom, the maitake is also known as hen-of-the-woods. Loved by chefs and health nuts alike, these earthy treasures can be roasted and tossed into salads or soups.

ROASTED MAITAKES

1 pound maitake mushrooms

1 tablespoon tamari

2 tablespoons grapeseed oil

Preheat the oven to 400°F. Gently toss the mushrooms into a bowl with the tamari and oil until coated. Spread the mushrooms onto a baking sheet in a single layer. After 5 minutes, flip the mushrooms, cook 5 to 7 more minutes until golden brown and serve.

MAKES 3 CUPS

Summer's stone fruits are a gift from God, and this divine crumble makes a heavenly breakfast. Hallelujah.

STONE FRUIT CRUMBLE

½ cup buckwheat flour

½ cup coconut flour

½ cup coconut flakes

½ cup maple syrup

1 tablespoon coconut oil

½ teaspoon Himalayan pink salt, divided

3 cups chopped assorted stone fruits

1 tablespoon dried lavender

2 tablespoons coconut sugar

Juice of 1 lemon

½ teaspoon vanilla extract or ¼ vanilla bean

1 tablespoon arrowroot

Om Chantilly (page 264)

Preheat the oven to 350°F.

In a large mixing bowl, combine the buckwheat flour, coconut flour, coconut flakes, syrup, oil and ¼ teaspoon of the salt. Set aside.

In another large mixing bowl, combine the fruit, lavender, sugar, lemon juice, vanilla, arrowroot and the remaining ¼ teaspoon salt. Mix well to combine. Transfer to a medium size baking dish and top with the flour crumble. Bake for 20 minutes, then rotate, and bake for another 15 to 20 minutes, or until the top becomes golden brown and the filling starts to bubble up. Serve with Om Chantilly.

SERVES 6

Savory for breakfast, and one of our secrets for starting the day off right. Our summer favorite is Spanish gazpacho. Light and refreshing, we recommend making it the night before. Cindy likes to keep a jar in the fridge so the whole family can partake. Any time of day. Add some avocado and head outside.

GOOD MORNING GAZPACHO

3 pounds tomatoes, coarsely chopped

2 cucumbers, coarsely chopped

2 jalapeño or serrano peppers, seeded and coarsely chopped (wear plastic gloves when handling)

3 cloves garlic

2 tablespoons olive oil, plus more for serving

2 tablespoons apple cider vinegar or sherry vinegar

1 tablespoon salt

1 tablespoon Spanish paprika

1 avocado, pitted, peeled, and chopped, divided

Add the tomatoes, cucumbers, peppers and garlic to a high-speed blender or food processor. Blend until fairly liquid. Add the oil, vinegar, salt, paprika and half of the avocado, and blend again. Chill in the fridge. Pour into your favorite bowls, top with a drizzle of oil and the remaining avocado and enjoy. Adjust salt to taste.

SERVES 4

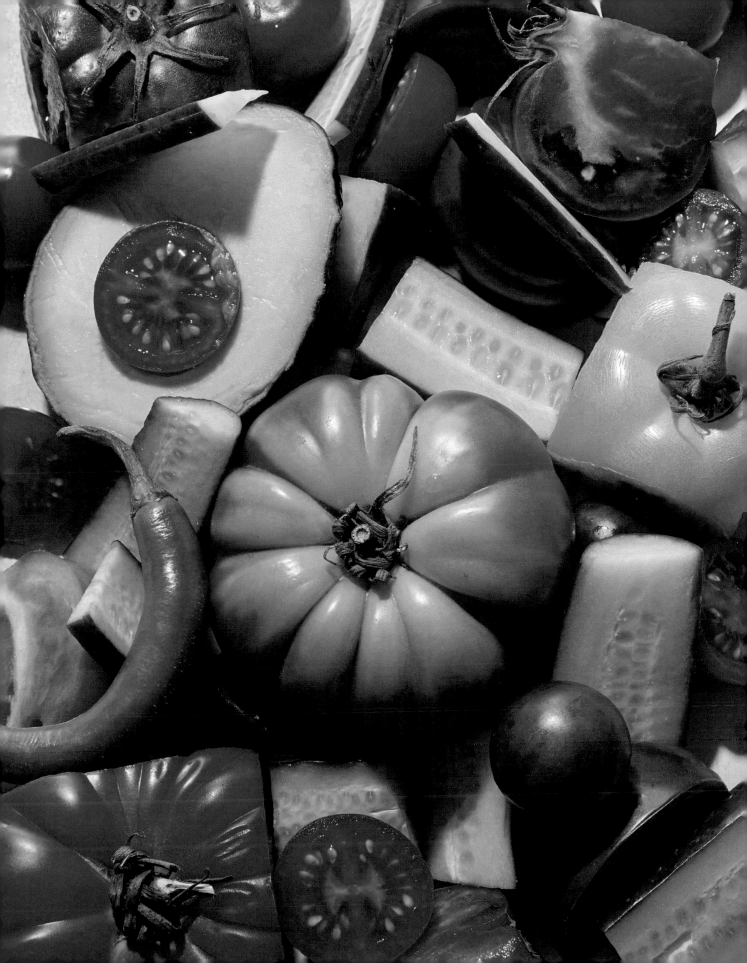

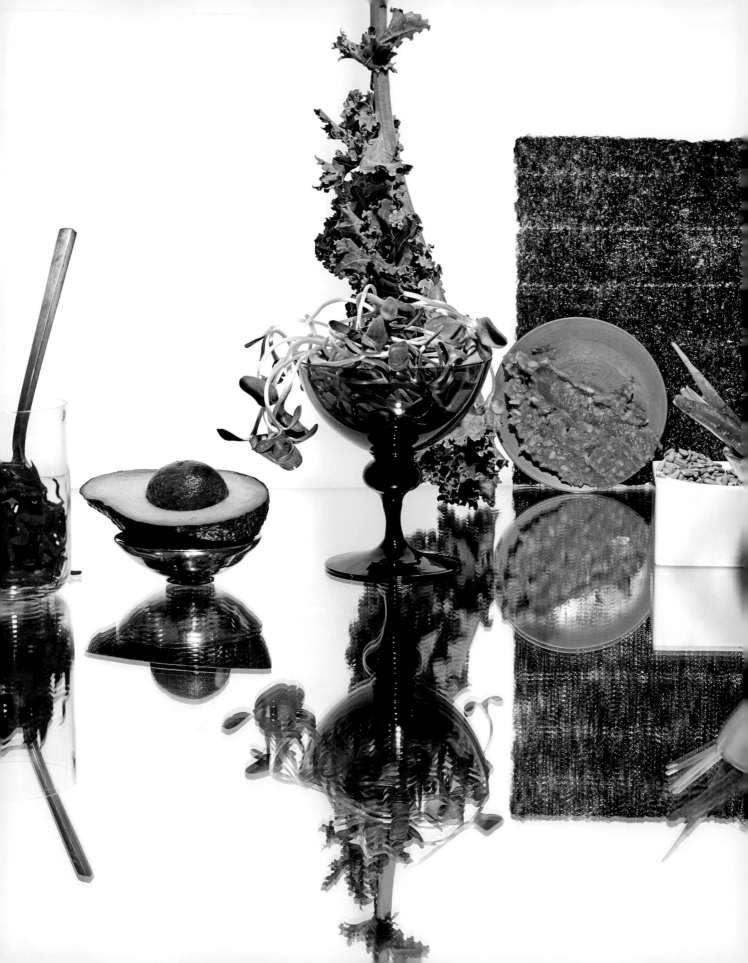

If you're having lunch or dinner at Kerrilynn and John's place in the summer, there's a good chance that you'll be introduced to the wrap. A staple in their home during the warmer months, they buy what looks good at the market and then head back and start rolling. Whatever you're craving, you're in good hands.

KERRILYNN'S GUIDE TO WRAPS

Nori sheets

Miso

Tahini

Sprouts (we like sunflower)

Fresh herbs

Microgreens

Sauerkraut

Cucumbers

Carrots

Avocados

Greens (we like romaine or kale)

Hemp seeds

Pepitas or sunflower seeds, seasoned or raw

The key here is getting all the ingredients together beforehand. Use mise en place to your advantage. Then, lay out the nori sheets, however many you are using, and consider this a little assembly line of health and deliciousness. Start with the sauce. Spread the miso or tahini directly on the wrap, lengthwise. Then, add the vegetables you want; this is your time to get creative, so pile them on. Just make sure to leave about 1 inch at the end so you can roll it up easily. Once all the fillings are in place, wet the edge of the nori and tightly roll the wrap up. You want them to be a bit wet so they hold together (if they're not, they will open up).

Heidi Swanson and her great blog, "101 Cookbooks", inspire many a meal in both of our kitchens. And, her sometimes rebellious approach to ingredients has taught us a lot (Nori Granola, anyone?). Her Heirloom Tomato Tart with its topping of raw summer tomatoes questions the need to bake. We took it a step (or three) further with a raw crust made of cauliflower instead of grains. The vibrant flavors of the garden come alive. This ode to Heidi is summer's perfect song.

SUMMER LOVING RAW TART

½ large head of cauliflower, florets only

¾ cup sunflower seeds

3 tablespoons flaxseed, ground

1 clove garlic, chopped

1 tablespoon coconut aminos or tamari

2 tablespoons nutritional yeast

¼ teaspoon Himalayan pink salt, plus more for sprinkling

Sunflower Ricotta (page 253)

Tonic Youth Pesto (page 49)

Heirloom tomatoes, sliced

Botija olives

Extra-virgin olive oil

Fresh basil

Prepare cauliflower "rice" by tossing the florets into a food processor and processing until broken down and ricelike (or by grating them on a large box grater). Measure out 2 cups and save the rest for another recipe. Then, combine the sunflower seeds, flaxseeds and garlic in the food processor and process until the seeds break down, about 15 seconds. Add in the 2 cups of cauliflower rice, coconut aminos or tamari, yeast and salt. Process until well-blended. Spread the dough out on a parchment-lined dehydrator sheet, about ¼ inch thick. Dehydrate at 145°F for 1 hour and then 115°F for an additional 5 to 6 hours, or until it is the consistency you like.

Add toppings, starting with a spread of ricotta and pesto and top with the tomatoes, olives, basil and a drizzle of oil. Top with a sprinkling of salt, and enjoy.

SERVES 4

NOTE: You can bake this at 300°F for 15 minutes, checking every 5 minutes thereafter. Remove from the oven when lightly golden brown and crispy.

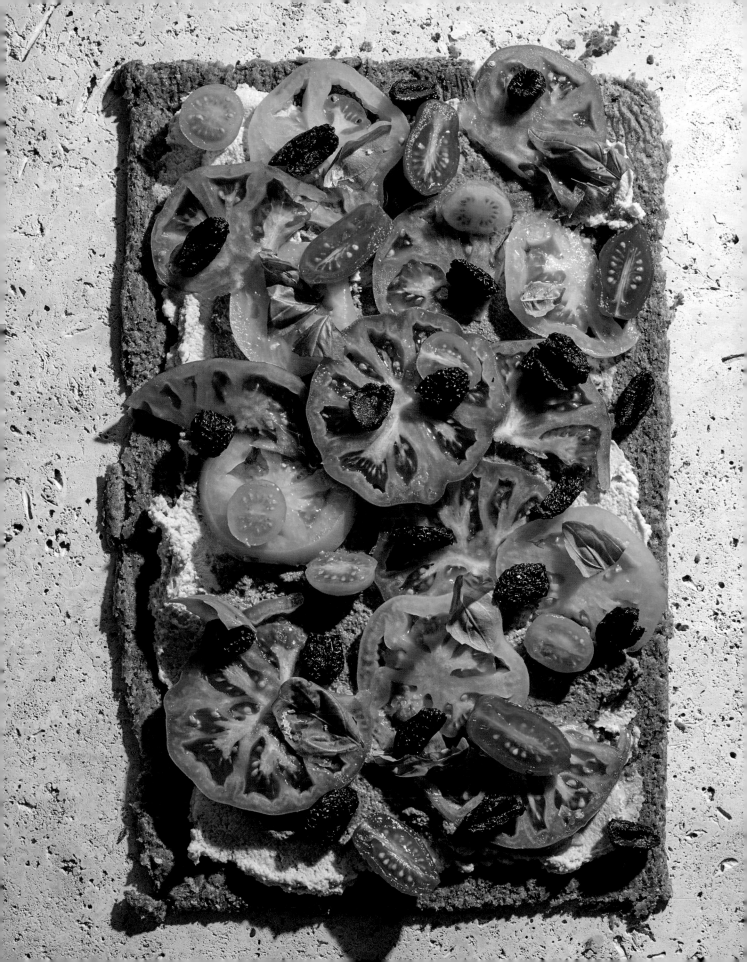

Our friend Nils introduced us to this dish years ago, and we've been dreaming about it ever since. Hailing from Contramar, the much-loved restaurant in Mexico City, theirs relies on tuna and mayonnaise, our version is CAP Beauty friendly and delicious. Bring Mexico home.

CONTRAMAR TORTILLAS

Corn tortillas
(4- to 5-inch diameter)

Coconut oil

1 cup coconut
mayonnaise

1 clove garlic, grated

1 teaspoon smoked
paprika

½ teaspoon ume plum
vinegar

1 cup smoked dulse

⅓ cup coconut aminos
or tamari

⅓ cup fresh lime juice

2 to 3 heirloom
tomatoes, sliced into
¼-inch-thick rounds

2 avocados, sliced
¼ inch thick

Fresh lime juice

Flaky sea salt

Preheat the oven to 400°F. Lay the tortillas onto a few parchment-lined baking sheets in a single layer. Lightly brush both sides with a small amount of melted coconut oil. Bake for 7 to 10 minutes, or until just starting to crisp up. Set aside.

Whisk together the mayonnaise, garlic, paprika and vinegar in a small mixing bowl or in a food processor. Set aside.

Reduce the oven temperature to the lowest setting. Spread the dulse out on a parchment-lined baking sheet and bake for about 5 minutes, or until brown and crisp. Set aside.

In a large mixing bowl, whisk together the aminos or tamari and lime juice. Add the tomatoes to the bowl and toss to combine. Allow to marinate for at least 5 minutes.

To assemble: Spread about 2 teaspoons of the mayonnaise onto each tortilla, followed by 2 slices of drained heirloom tomatoes. Then, sprinkle 1½ teaspoons of dulse followed by 2 to 3 slices of avocado. Top with lime juice and salt.

SERVES 4

A bright and elevated dish from our friend and acupuncturist, Frances Boswell, this fresh and briny raw salad makes a perfect hot weather meal atop a bowl of quinoa or brown rice. Keep it simple, fresh and light. Then, get outside.

THE QUICK PICK SALAD

1 cucumber, thinly sliced

2 carrots, sliced

1 scallion, thinly sliced into long strips

3 tablespoons apple cider vinegar

Several handfuls lentil, mung bean and/or chickpea sprouts

Handful of cilantro, stems removed

Handful of mint, stems removed

1 tablespoon tamari

Large dash of sesame oil

2 tablespoons sesame seeds

Cooked quinoa or brown rice

Sunflower, pumpkin or hemp seeds

Combine the cucumber, carrots and scallion in a medium mixing bowl. Add the vinegar, toss well and let stand for about 15 minutes. Add the sprouts, cilantro, mint, tamari and oil. Sprinkle in the sesame seeds. Serve over the quinoa or rice with a scattering of sunflower, pumpkin or hemp seeds.

SERVES 1 OR 2

Aloha, little poke. This classic dish from Hawaii is having a moment. And, for good reason. The delicious combination of fresher than fresh fish brings vacation to you. Our version taps into the neverending power of plants. Top with greens or eat it straight from your favorite bowl. This is island living at its best.

OUR WAY POKE

1 scallion, sliced thinly

½ sweet onion, finely diced

1½ tablespoons tamari or coconut aminos

1 tablespoon fresh lemon juice

1 teaspoon honey or coconut sugar

1 teaspoon grated ginger

2 teaspoons toasted sesame oil

1 tablespoon black sesame seeds, toasted

2 cups ripe papaya chunks (½ inch)

¼ cup hijiki

Cauliflower Coconut Rice (page 214)

GARNISHES (OPTIONAL):
Sliced avocado

Shiso, cilantro, mint

Scallions, sliced on the bias

Toasted macadamia nuts

Holy Herbs Schichimi (page 266)

Red pepper flakes

Lime wedges

Whisk together the scallion, onion, tamari or aminos, lemon juice, honey or sugar, ginger, oil and sesame seeds in a large mixing bowl. Add the papaya and mix well. Transfer to the refrigerator and let sit in marinade overnight.

Soak the hijiki in warm water to rehydrate for 5 to 10 minutes. Drain and squeeze out any excess moisture. Add the hijiki to the bowl of papaya, and mix well.

Mound ½ to ¾ cup of cauliflower rice on a plate, top with ½ to ¾ cup of the papaya and add any garnishes you desire.

SERVES 4

NOTE: You can make a spicy poke sauce by combining ½ cup coconut mayonnaise with 1 tablespoon lacto-fermented hot sauce and ½ teaspoon sweetener.

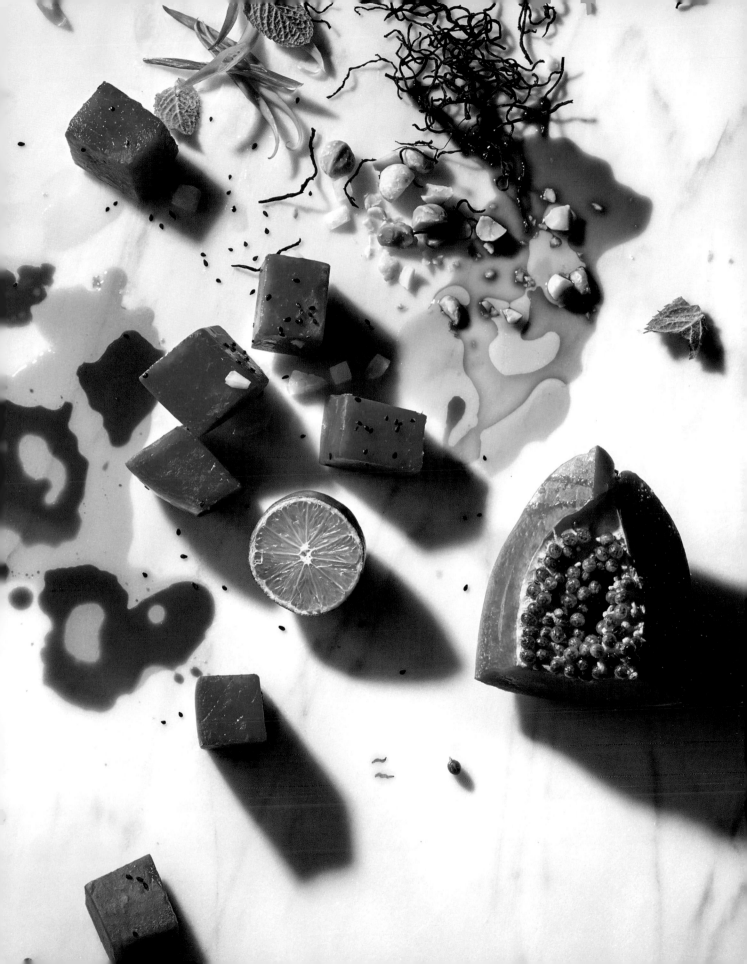

Africa's answer to guacamole, tomatoes, avocados and chiles are tossed together with bits of *injera*, a sour Ethiopian bread made from fermented teff flour. We fell in love with Fit Fit at our friend Pierre's West Village restaurant, Injera, home to many a CAP Beauty dinner. We often share the room with Pierre at Sky Ting Yoga and love his commitment to health, sport and delicious food.

PIERROT'S FIT FIT

1 serrano chile

1 Injera (page 270), torn into 1-inch pieces, plus more for serving

1 avocado, pitted and chopped

1 pint cherry tomatoes, halved

1 small red onion, chopped

Big pinch of Himalayan pink salt

Olive oil

Juice of 1 lemon

Mince the chile, removing the seeds if you like a milder dish. Add half to a mixing bowl with the injera, avocado, tomatoes, onion and salt. Drizzle with oil and lemon juice, and toss to combine. Taste and add the remaining chile, if desired. Serve with additional injera.

SERVES 2 TO 4

Take it higher. A combination of our favorite seeds and fruits keeps us fueled for the day. One of our favorite snacks for a long day spent out, bring them on the road for a healthy and filling snack, and elevate yourself.

ALTITUDE MIX

1 cup pepitas

½ cup sunflower seeds

½ cup cacao nibs

¾ cup goji berries

1 cup large coconut flakes

Put all ingredients in a medium mixing bowl, and stir to combine.

MAKES 3 CUPS

Kerrilynn's husband is the master of snacks, and his take on one of our favorite snack foods, Sprouties, is a testament to his genius. His addition of Ethiopian berbere and apple cider vinegar uplevels them, while adding a bit of spice and tang. Crunchy and addictive, these seeds are great on top of a salad or eaten straight up. We like them any time of day. Any way.

JOHN'S BRIGHT, LIGHT PEPITAS

1 cup pepitas

1 cup apple cider vinegar

1 tablespoon Berbere (page 267) or crushed chile blend

4 tablespoons nutritional yeast

½ cup small coconut flakes

1 teaspoon Himalayan pink salt

In a medium bowl, soak the pepitas in the vinegar overnight. Strain, and reserve the vinegar for another batch, if desired. In a small bowl, combine the Berbere or chile blend, yeast, coconut and salt. Pour over the pepitas, making sure to cover and distribute the mixture evenly. Put in the dehydrator for 18 to 24 hours at 118°F (check at 18 hours, and, if not crisp, keep dehydrating). Alternatively, bake in a 350°F oven for 1 hour, stirring often.

SERVES MANY

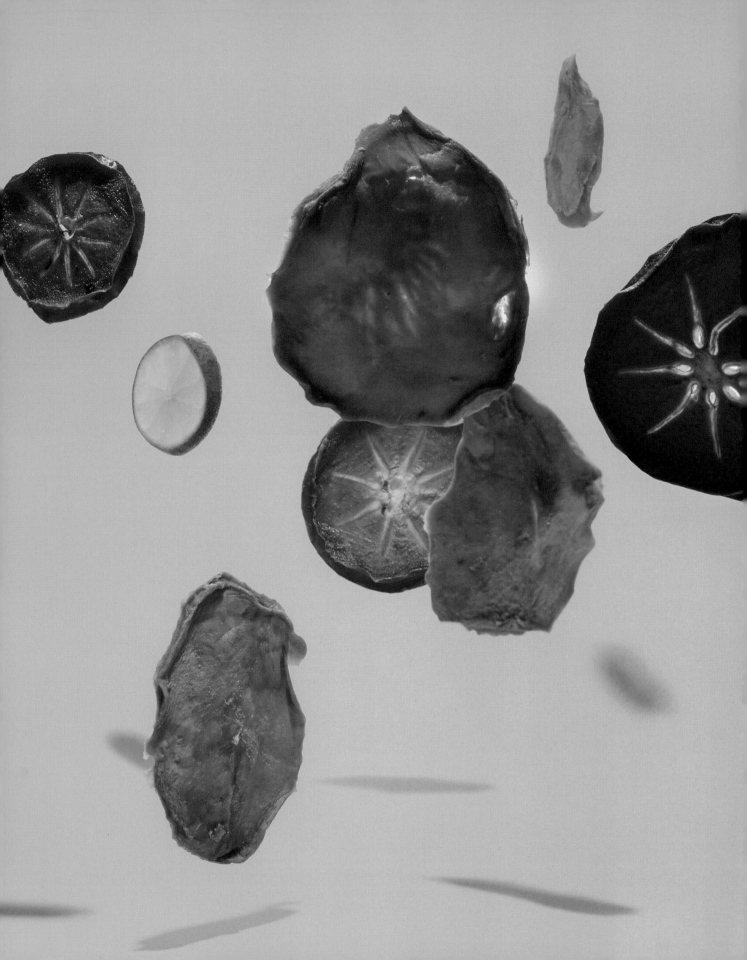

Street food done right. One of our favorite snacks, this treat tastes just like summer: spicy, tart and juicy. Put your bathing suit on, and get yourself to the beach. Your towel is waiting.

MEXICALI MANGO

2 cups dried mango

1½ cups fresh lime juice

1 bunch of fresh mint

Place the mango in a medium bowl and cover with the lime juice and mint. Soak overnight. Strain and place on dehydrator tray. Set the dehydrator at 118°F and cook for 18 to 24 hours. Alternatively, you can bake in the oven at the lowest setting for 1 hour.

SERVES MANY

Lighten up. This summery version of a high hippie staple swaps heavier chickpeas for raw fresh zucchini and the cooling bite of mint.

GARDEN BOX HUMMUS

2 zucchinis, halved lengthwise

1 teaspoon coconut or olive oil

1 small garlic clove

¼ cup tahini

¼ cup mint leaves

¼ teaspoon turmeric

3 tablespoons fresh lemon juice

1½ tablespoons olive oil

Freshly ground black pepper

Preheat the oven to 400°F.

Place the zucchini, cut-side down, on a parchment-lined baking sheet and rub all over with coconut or olive oil. Roast until tender and lightly browned, about 30 minutes. Set aside.

In a food processor, combine the garlic, tahini, mint, turmeric, lemon juice and 1½ tablespoons olive oil, and process until well-combined. Chop up the reserved zucchini and add it to the food processor. Process until well-combined, scraping down the sides, if necessary. Transfer to a bowl, and add pepper.

MAKES ABOUT 2½ CUPS

We all scream for ice cream. "Nice Cream," that is. Sultry summer evenings and beachy afternoons beg for a trip to the ice cream parlor. So, we've remade the classic sundae for the hazy, lazy high days of summer. Treat the kids. Treat yourself. Indulge in summer, CAP Beauty style. We've included our favorite toppings, but add whatever you like to customize your sundae.

HIGH SUMMER SUNDAE

½ cup Aquafaba (page 261), room temperature

½ cup plus 1 tablespoon coconut sugar

2 teaspoons vanilla extract or 1 vanilla bean

½ cup coconut cream

½ teaspoon Himalayan pink salt

1 cup cherries, pitted and halved

¼ cup pureed sea buckthorn berries* or orange juice

⅓ cup coconut oil

½ cup raw cacao powder

Fresh summer fruit

Banana

Toasted coconut flakes

Om Chantilly (page 264)

In a mixer bowl, beat the aquafaba on high-speed until stiff peaks form, about 10 minutes. With the machine still running, slowly pour in ½ cup of the sugar, 1 tablespoon at a time. Continue to beat. Add in the vanilla and coconut cream, and continue to beat until thoroughly combined, about 5 more minutes. Scrape down the sides of the bowl, as necessary. Transfer to a storage container and place in the freezer to chill overnight.

Over medium-low heat, gently heat the salt, cherries, sea buckthorn puree or orange juice and the remaining 1 tablespoon of the sugar in a small saucepan, and stir until the sugar dissolves. Allow to cool, then refrigerate.

Meanwhile, heat the oil in a double boiler. Whisk in the cacao. Allow to cool for 5 minutes. Use immediately or store in the refrigerator. It will harden if stored in the refrigerator, so you will have to gently rewarm before using.

Remove the nice cream from the freezer and scoop into serving bowls, and top with the fruit, banana and coconut flakes, then add the chocolate sauce, Om Chantilly, and cherry sauce.

SERVES 6

NOTE: Before freezing the "nice" cream, try adding ½ cup cacao powder, 2 tablespoons finely ground coffee or ½ cup strawberry puree.

You can buy sea buckthorn berry puree at capbeauty.com, or through other online retailers.

Shake your tree. And, when the peaches fall, make pie. This sweet and surprising tart has just the right amount of bite.

PEACHY PIE

1 cup raw almonds

½ cup raw oats, plus more if needed

Pinch of Himalayan pink salt

¾ cup medjool dates, pitted

1 tablespoon coconut oil, plus more if needed

1 tablespoon apple cider vinegar or fresh lemon juice

1 tablespoon honey or maple syrup

3 ripe summer peaches

½ cup Om Chantilly (page 264)

1 teaspoon ground or finely minced fresh ginger

1 tablespoon raw honey (optional)

Spoonful of bee pollen (optional)

Pulse the almonds in the bowl of a food processor until they reach the consistency of a coarse meal. Add the oats and salt, and pulse to combine. Add the dates and oil, and pulse until sticky and combined. You may need to pause and scrape down the sides a few times during this process. If the dough is too dry, add a touch more oil. If it's too sticky, add more oats. Press the crust into the bottom and up the sides of a tart or pie pan, or use a springform pan. Set in the fridge to cool.

Add the vinegar or lemon juice and the honey or syrup to a small mixing bowl and whisk to combine. Peel and slice two of the peaches, and add to the bowl. Toss to combine. Set aside to macerate.

Peel and chop the remaining peach and place it in a high-speed blender along with the whipped cream, ginger and honey (if using). Blend until smooth. Spread a layer of the whipped cream mixture onto the pie crust and top with the peaches. Store in the fridge until ready to serve. Garnish with bee pollen (if using).

SERVES 10

BEE POLLEN

Nectar of the gods. We eat this like candy and sprinkle it on desserts, in tonic drinks, on fresh fruit and in smoothies. Rich in antiviral and antibacterial compounds, and high in vitamins and minerals, this sweet treat gets us buzzing every time.

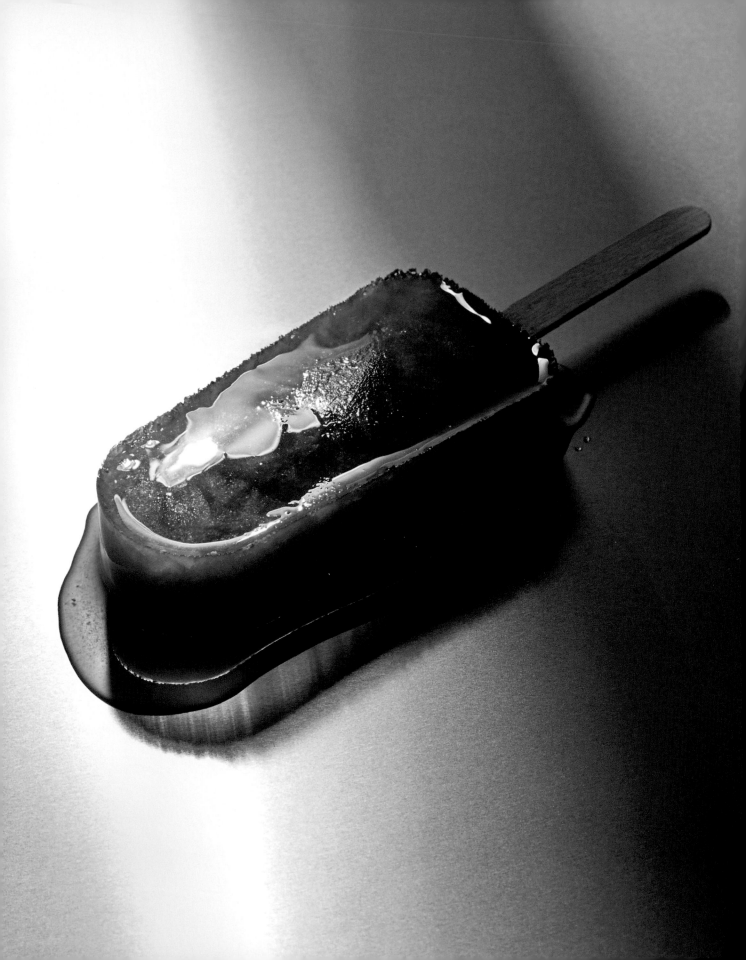

Western herbalists use elderflower as an anti-inflammatory and antiseptic to fight common colds, flu and even allergies. Mixologists everywhere use elderflower to impart its fragrant floral notes to cocktails and tonics. These elegant ice pops are just what the doctor (and bartender) ordered.

ELDERFLOWER POWER POPS

½ cup coconut sugar

3½ cups filtered water

¼ cup dried elderflower or ½ cup fresh

½ cup fresh lemon juice

1 tablespoon lemon zest

Place the sugar and ½ cup of the water in a small saucepan. Gently heat and whisk until the sugar has dissolved. Allow to cool. Meanwhile, put the remaining 3 cups of water, the elderflower, lemon juice and lemon zest into a large jar. Use only the blossoms as the stems, stalks, twigs and leaves are toxic. Add the sugar water. Refrigerate for 24 hours and then strain. Discard the zest and elderflower. Pour the infused liquid into ice pop molds and freeze for at least 6 hours.

MAKES 6 TO 8 POPS

NOTE: Add ½ cup roughly chopped herbs, such as mint, lemon balm/verbena or sorrel, into the molds before freezing.

Cindy has become known for her unique and much loved chocolates that she regularly (not regularly enough!) brings to the office. And, this summery version with coconut butter, blueberries, tocotrienols and deep blue bilberry powder is the most recent addition to her repertoire. Equally good for breakfast, these delicious bites deliver healthy fat, vitamins D and E and antioxidant power. A case of the blues never tasted so good.

BLUE VELVETS

1 pint blueberries

½ cup tocotrienols

2 tablespoons bilberry powder

Juice of ¼ small lemon

⅓ cup coconut oil

1 (16-ounce) jar coconut butter

2 tablespoons maple syrup (optional)

Add the blueberries, tocotrienols, bilberry powder, lemon juice and 1 tablespoon of the coconut oil to a high-speed blender or food processor and puree. Set aside. In the top of a double boiler (or in a metal mixing bowl set atop a saucepan of simmering water) gently heat the remaining coconut oil, the butter and syrup (if using). Remove from the heat and stir in the blueberry mixture. Pour into standard-size chocolate molds, and chill. When firm, turn them out and store in a lidded glass container in the fridge.

MAKES 24

Reese's gets a makeover. Dark raw chocolate wrapped around maca (a South American root believed to increase libido, fertility and good vibes) and almond butter conjures up the sweets of our childhood, but leaves us feeling high and happy. Your inner child will thank you.

SUPERIORITY CUPS

⅔ cup plus 1 tablespoon coconut oil

1 cup raw cacao powder

⅓ cup maple syrup

2 tablespoons maca

¼ teaspoon Himalayan pink salt

2 to 3 tablespoons unsalted creamy almond or seed butter

Line a mini muffin pan with baking cups. Melt the oil gently in a small saucepan over low heat. Turn off the heat and stir in the cacao, syrup, maca and salt. Spoon ½ teaspoon of the mixture into each baking cup. Reserve the remaining chocolate. Place the muffin pan in the freezer, and remove after 15 to 20 minutes, or when the chocolate is firm. Scoop ¼ teaspoon of the almond or seed butter onto each chocolate round, pressing down gently to flatten, making sure that the butter remains centered. Gently reheat the reserved chocolate, then pour enough of the melted chocolate to completely cover the almond or seed butter. Place in the freezer again for 30 minutes, or until the chocolate is firm. Keep refrigerated.

MAKES 12

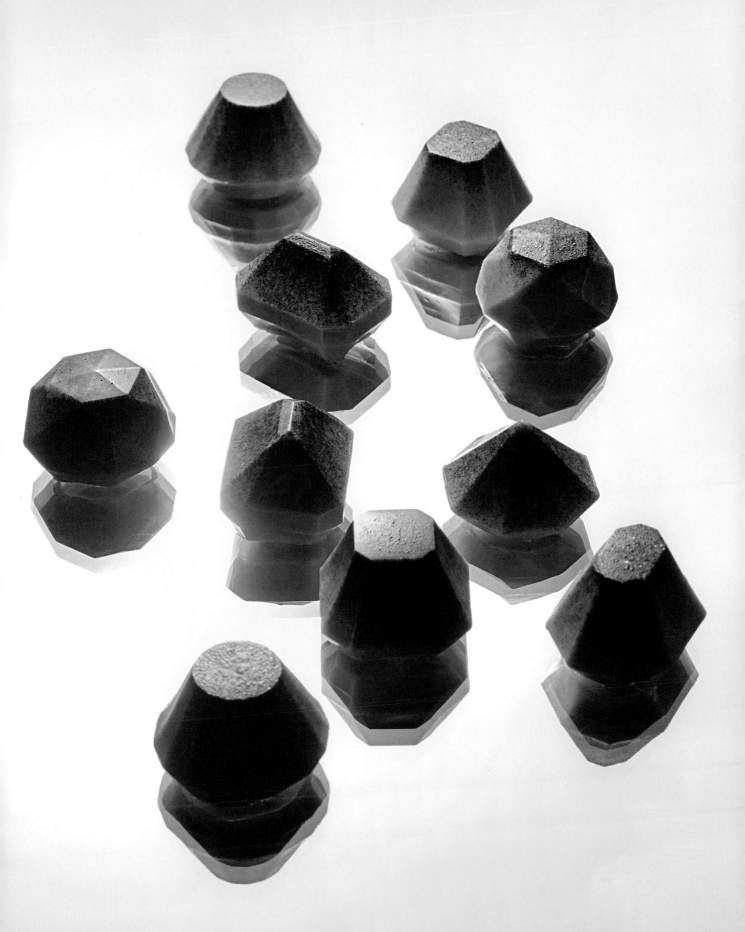

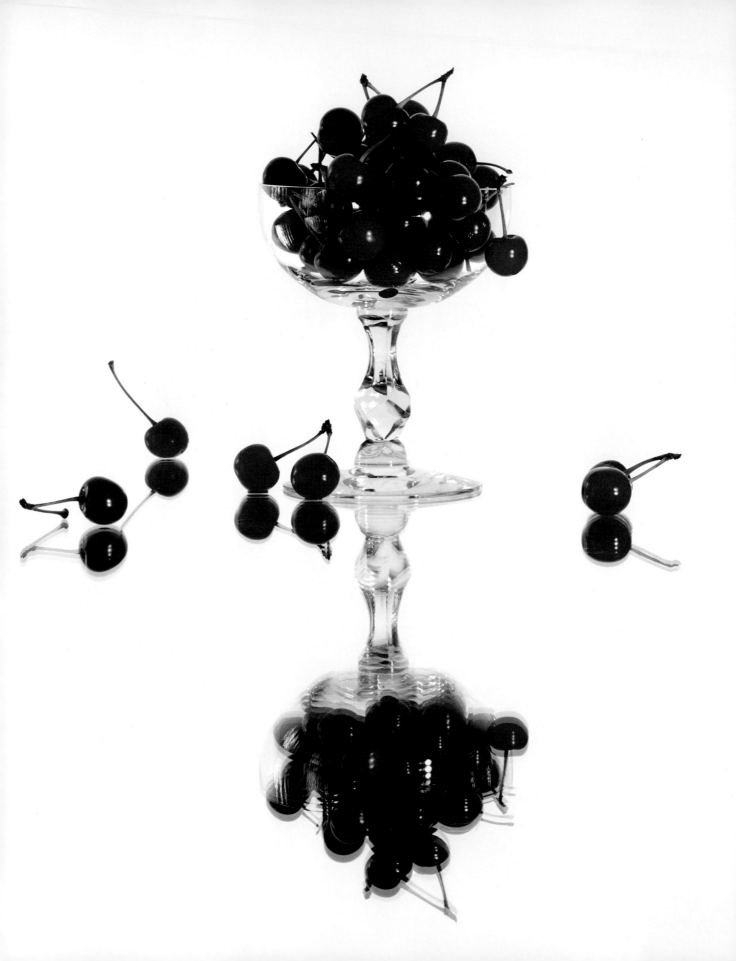

One of the last remaining truly seasonal ingredients, sour cherries are available for just a few short weeks at the height of summer. Don't let them pass you by. These bright red gems are beautifully tart and alive with flavor. Cindy's Sour Cherry Pie is a summer tradition, but, in recent years, it's been upleveled. A perfect way to celebrate America the beautiful.

SMART TART PIE

2 tablespoons ground chia seeds

6 tablespoons filtered water

2 cups coconut flour

2 cups brown rice flour

4 tablespoons coconut sugar, plus more for sprinkling

¾ teaspoon Himalayan pink salt

2 tablespoons coconut oil, melted, plus more as needed

3 cups tart cherries, halved and pitted

Zest of 1 lemon

1 teaspoon vanilla extract or ½ vanilla bean)

2 tablespoons arrowroot

Om Chantilly (page 264)

Preheat the oven to 350°F. In a small bowl, combine the chia seeds and water and let sit for 10 minutes to thicken. In a large mixing bowl, whisk together the coconut flour, rice flour, 2 tablespoons of the sugar and ½ teaspoon of the salt. Add in the oil and chia, and mix well. Refrigerate for 15 to 30 minutes, then divide the dough into two. Grease an 8-inch pie pan with 1 teaspoon coconut oil. Press half of the dough into the pie pan, covering the bottom and sides of the dish. Prick the dough with a fork, then bake for 10 to 15 minutes, or until lightly browned. Set aside. Place the remaining half of the dough between two layers of parchment paper and roll it out into a circle 9 inches in diameter. Place it in the refrigerator or freezer to chill.

Place the cherries, the remaining 2 tablespoons of the sugar, the lemon zest, vanilla, arrowroot and the remaining ¼ teaspoon of salt in a medium saucepan. Place over medium heat. Bring to a boil and reduce to a simmer. Gently cook for about 30 minutes, or until jammy in consistency.

Place the cherry filling in the pie pan. Gently place the top crust of dough over the filling and secure it by crimping edges (using the tines of a fork is helpful here). Brush the top with a bit of melted coconut oil and a sprinkle of sugar. Cut a few holes in the top using a knife or a cookie cutter, so that the filling can breathe during baking, and place the pie dish on a cookie sheet to avoid spills. Bake for 30 to 40 minutes, or until the crust is golden brown. Allow to cool before enjoying. Serve with Om Chantilly.

SERVES 6 TO 8

The highest vibrational plant we know, rose infuses this classic comfort food, lending a Persian twist and a fragrant perfumed profile. A magical dessert for a night under the stars.

PERSIAN ROSE RICE PUDDING

1 cup brown rice

1 15-ounce can full-fat coconut milk

2 tablespoons filtered water, plus more as needed

2 tablespoons dried edible organic rose petals, crushed

Seeds of 6 cardamom pods, crushed

½ teaspoon vanilla extract (or ¼ vanilla bean)

2 tablespoons honey or coconut nectar

¼ teaspoon Himalayan pink salt

Pistachios

Rose petals

In a medium saucepan, combine all ingredients and cook over medium low heat until the liquid has been absorbed and the rice has cooked through. Add more water, if necessary. Allow to cool and transfer to the refrigerator to chill. When ready to serve, divide between four bowls and top with the pistachios and rose petals.

SERVES 4

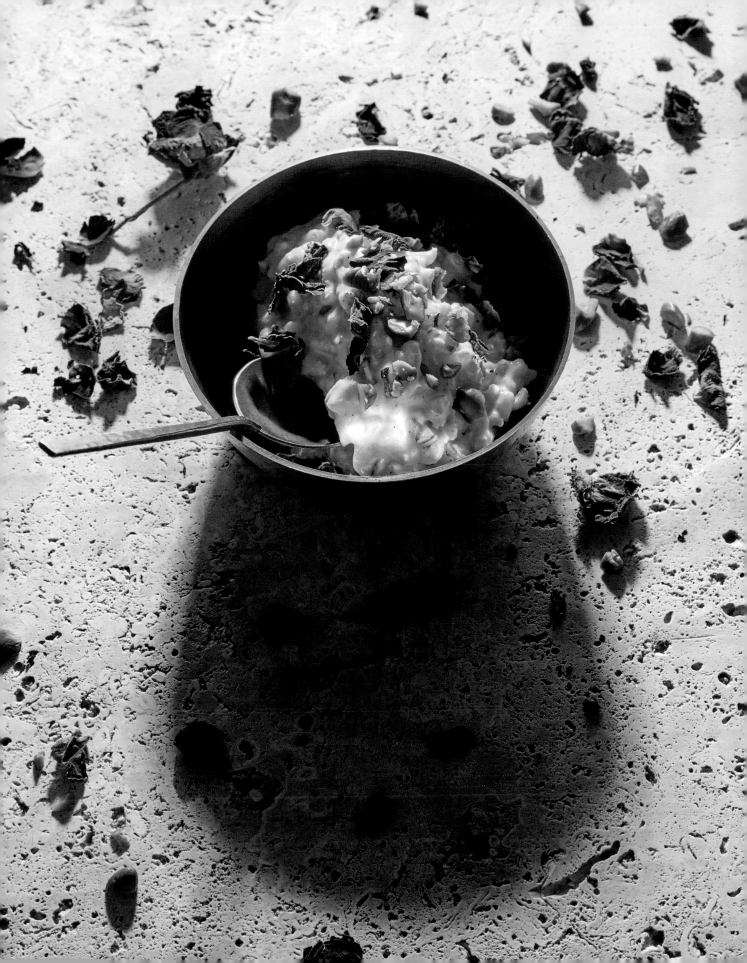

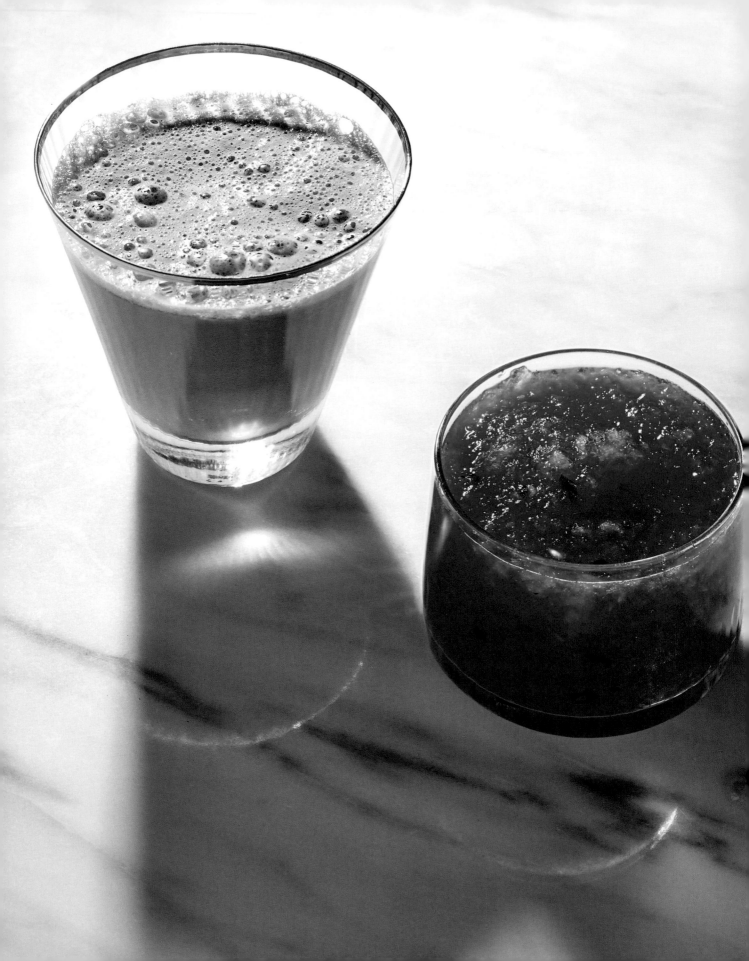

This elevated drink relies on protein-heavy tiger nuts and fragrant hibiscus to deliver an elegant take on one of our favorite Mexican street drinks, the classic horchata. Hibiscus ice cubes lend their floral notes to the earthy, sweet and prebiotic-heavy tiger nuts, resulting in a pink tower of power. Feel the roar.

HIBISCUS HORCHATA

1 cup tiger nuts

8 cups filtered water, divided

½ cup dried hibiscus flowers

¼ cup honey

½ teaspoon vanilla powder or 1 teaspoon vanilla extract

Using two separate containers, soak the nuts in 4 cups of water and the flowers in 4 cups of water in the refrigerator for 24 hours.

Strain the nuts and discard the soaking liquid. Transfer them to a high-speed blender. Strain the hibiscus liquid into the blender, discarding or composting the flowers. Blend on high until the mixture is completely smooth, about 1 to 2 minutes. Strain the mixture through a cheesecloth. Stir in the honey and vanilla, and serve over ice.

SERVES 4

A love letter to leisurely, summer days, this refreshing and supremely hydrating drink is a new favorite. Watermelon spiked with mint and lime offers a new take on a slushie, one that's supremely satisfying, good for you and pink. A trifecta of power.

MINTED MELON ICE

6 cups watermelon, seeded and chopped

Juice of 1 lime

2 tablespoons goji berries

⅓ cup mint leaves

2 dates, seeded

2 cups ice

Place the watermelon, lime juice, berries, mint and dates in a blender and process at high speed until smooth. Add the ice and blend until broken down (using a blender tamper to break up the ice chunks is helpful).

SERVES 4

NOTE: Makes a great summertime High Vibe cocktail with ¼ ounce tequila in each glass, finished with a Himalayan pink salt rim!

Get high and hot on this libido boosting cocktail of love. Pine pollen increases desire, while bitters soothe inflammation, creating a perfect environment for a night to remember. Bottoms up, buttercup.

PINE POLLEN FIZZ

2 cups sparkling mineral water (we like Gerolsteiner or Mountain Valley)

2 tablespoons pureed sea buckthorn berries*

1 teaspoon pine pollen

Pour the mineral water in your favorite glasses, leaving some room at the top, as the pine pollen can be fizzy. Add the sea buckthorn and pine pollen, and stir to combine. The pine pollen has a tendency to clump up, so make sure to stir thoroughly. Enjoy!

SERVES 2

You can buy sea buckthorn berry puree at capbeauty.com, or through other online retailers.

Inspired by many a black and tan from the pub, a previous elixir of choice, consider this the friendlier, more elevated version. Long-steeped chaga (the king of medicinal mushrooms known for its anti-inflammatory and skin supporting properties) is brimming with benefits for the body and mind, and seed milk offers up the creaminess you expect from the classic bar drink. Bottoms up. To your health.

CHAGA BLACK AND TAN

12 tablespoons chaga

12 cups filtered water, plus more if needed

1 cup Power-Up Seed Milk (page 251)

Add the chaga and water to a large pot. Bring to a boil, then reduce the heat and let simmer for 6 hours. Check the water levels from time to time. Make sure that the liquid doesn't get too low. It will evaporate some, but you want about 2 cups of chaga concentrate.

Add ½ tablespoon chaga concentrate to your favorite glass and pour the milk on top. Stir to combine. Enjoy!

MAKES ENOUGH FOR 32 DRINKS

Cindy's daughter Sally is obsessed with all things pink. And, luckily, this pretty pink drink is as delicious as it is loaded with nutritious whole foods. It's great for kids and adults alike. Have it for breakfast or as an after beach or after dinner snack. For a creamier version, use nut or coconut milk, or for a lighter, fresher take, use coconut water. And, if you like a bit of bite, spike it with a dash of ume vinegar, but omit the salt.

THINK PINK STRAWBERRY MILK

1 cup brazil nut milk, coconut milk, or coconut water

4 to 5 ripe strawberries

1 tablespoon tocotrienols

1 teaspoon coconut butter

Pinch of Himalayan pink salt (omit if using vinegar)

Dash of ume vinegar (optional)

Add all the ingredients to a high-speed blender and blend until smooth. Serve cold.

SERVES 1

AUTUMN

AN INTRO TO AUTUMN: BACK TO EARTH

Ground down to fly high. After the high life of summer, we greet autumn with open hearts and open arms. autumn marks a return to home and to ourselves, a time to reconnect. For many, this is a season of starting anew, a time to create and a time to manifest. Settle in, and welcome the quiet. It's all around you.

The recipes and grounding rituals shared here help us connect to the planet and to our inner guides. Quietude, solitude and deep self care support us through the seasonal shift. Look inward to find your light for the days ahead.

THE AUTUMN SKIN PROGRAM

PERFORM: Once or twice daily, masking once a week or scrubbing 1 or 2 times per week

WHAT YOU'LL NEED: A cleanser, toner and oil or moisturizer, plus an exfoliant

DURATION: 5 to 10 minutes

After summer's salty and sunny good times, we look to uncover healthy and happy skin. Layers of sunscreen, days at the beach and sweating it out can leave your skin in less than pristine condition.

At this time of year, we add mild to deep exfoliation to our skincare programs. This will depend on your level of sensitivity, your moon cycle and what's on the agenda.

The enzymes in pumpkin and honey work wonders to create an effective and nutrient-dense exfoliating mask. Others may prefer a physical exfoliant, such as a scrub. We don't recommend exfoliating before an important date or an evening out, as your skin may need some time to recover. And, if you know that you're extremely sensitive, skip this altogether and choose a honey mask instead.

HOW TO DO IT: In the autumn, follow your standard morning and evening skincare routines, adding an appropriate exfoliant to the program. For some, this is a mask, and, for others, this is a manual scrub. Always exfoliate in the evening, so your skin has time to rest and recover.

If masking, look for products with active botanicals, such as pumpkin and other fruit enzymes. Pineapple is excellent, too. Before you use any new product, but especially with enzymatic exfoliants, test a patch on your inner wrist and monitor it for any reaction. On your clean face, apply a thin layer of mask. Monitor your skin for its level of heat, and, if you feel like your skin is reacting strongly, remove it at once. Be mindful that these masks can be powerful. They reveal beautiful skin, but it's important not to overdo it. Let your skin breathe afterward. Skip any active serums until the next night, and revel in your perfect new canvas.

Or, make your own simple-yet-effective version at home. One of our favorite beauty routines is to apply manuka honey to the skin for 5 to 10 minutes.

If using a manual scrub, start with clean skin. Use gentle circular motions, and remember to keep your face damp. Continue for up to a minute, then rinse. Follow with a rich and gentle moisturizer, but, again, skip any active serums until the following evening.

THE RITUALS: GROUNDING DOWN

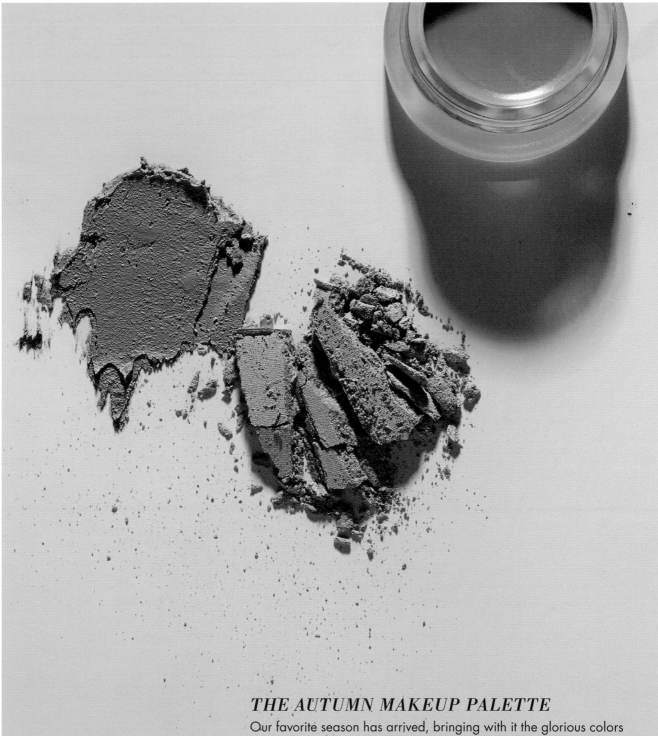

THE AUTUMN MAKEUP PALETTE

Our favorite season has arrived, bringing with it the glorious colors of autumn. Look no further than the turning leaves for inspiration. Copper, rust, bronze and tawny browns create a nature made foundation and a perfect canvas for hints of deep teal, rich magenta or hunter green. We also love to add a shocking yellow. Pair it all with a nude lip, and set the town ablaze.

HAIR MASKS

PERFORM:
Once a week

WHAT YOU'LL NEED:
For dry hair, a
treatment oil or cold
pressed coconut oil.
For oily hair, apple
cider vinegar, raw
honey, a lemon or
cup of brewed
hibiscus tea, a small
mixing bowl and a
wide-toothed wooden
comb or brush

DURATION:
30 minutes
to overnight

Sun, sand and surf can lead to ravaged locks. And, whether you swing dry and damaged or limp and oily, a mask can restore health and shine. Greet autumn with healthy hair, by introducing these simple masks into your weekly routine.

HOW TO DO IT: For dry or damaged hair, apply the oil directly to your dry scalp. Massage in and work the oil down through the length of your hair, making sure that the ends are saturated. Your comb will help with this. You may need to add more oil to the mid-sections and ends. How much you need will depend on the length of your hair. Hair should be just coated, not superwet. Wrap your hair in a towel, and leave it on for 1 hour to overnight. This is a great time to take a bath, as the humidity will benefit the process. When ready, shampoo and condition normally.

For oily hair, combine ¼ cup apple cider vinegar (ACV), the juice of 1 lemon and 1 tablespoon raw honey in a small mixing bowl. You can substitute 2 tablespoons brewed 100 percent hibiscus tea for the lemon. In Ayurveda, hibiscus is known to encourage thicker hair growth as well as condition the hair. Mix with a small whisk and apply to damp hair, using your comb to distribute. Leave on your hair for just 30 minutes.

Again, this is a perfect time for a bath. Otherwise, wrap your hair in a towel. When ready, shampoo hair normally to remove.

THE AUTUMN BATH

PERFORM: Once
or twice a week

WHAT YOU'LL NEED:
Organic apple cider
vinegar

DURATION:
20 to 30 minutes

An apple a day. This season calls to mind one of our favorite bathing rituals, the apple cider vinegar bath. This health food store staple, known for its alkalizing ways, does wonders for the skin and beyond. A natural antibacterial, this vinegar clears up fungus-based skin conditions and restores pH balance to the skin. What goes on your skin goes in your body, and a vinegar bath can also help with digestion and relieve inflammation and joint pain. Since we absorb its nutrients, notably the elusive B vitamins, vitamin C and trace minerals, this bath works on an inner and outer beauty level. It's no wonder that we sing its praises. Skin will feel moisturized and clarified, and apple cider vinegar does wonders for hair health, too. Take the plunge.

HOW TO DO IT: Fill your tub with hot water, and add 1 to 2 cups of the vinegar. Soak for 20 to 30 minutes, or until the water cools. Use a washcloth, if you like, and don't be afraid to get your hair wet. Some like a shower afterward (especially if you've gotten your hair wet), but others recommend letting the vinegar dry on your skin.

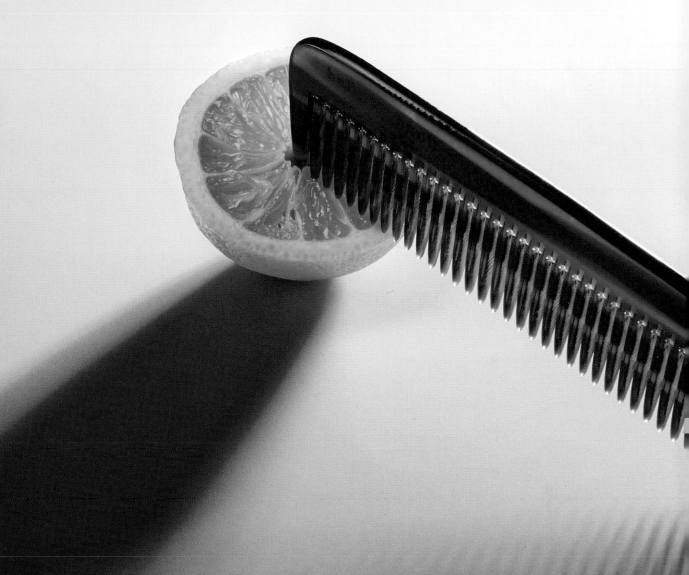

AUTUMN PRODUCT RECOMMENDATIONS

CLEANSER: Wedderspoon Manuka Honey, Tata Harper Regenerating Cleanser, One Love Organics Vitamin B Active Moisture Cleansing Oil

HYDROSOL: Mūn Anarose Hydrating Rose Toner, Julisis Silver Cistus Toner Night, The Beauty Chef Probiotic Skin Refiner

MOISTURIZER: Kahina Giving Beauty Facial Lotion, Max and Me Sweet Serenity Balm, Shiva Rose Pearl Rose Face Cream

EXFOLIANT: May Lindstrom The Clean Dirt, S. W. Basics Cream Scrub, Odacité Jojoba Beads Exfoliant

OTHER GOOD STUFF: Leahlani Honey Love Three in One, Living Libations Green + Papaya Lime AHA Mask, Butter Elixir Lip

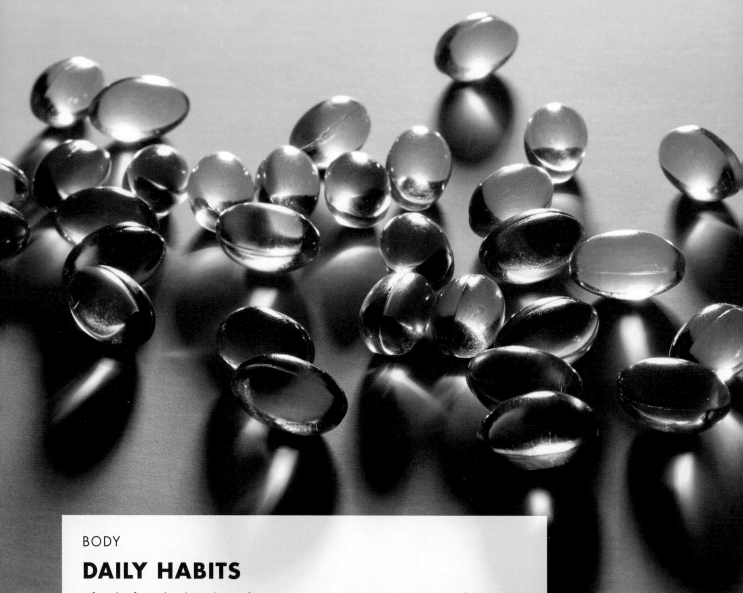

BODY

DAILY HABITS

After the freewheeling days of summer, we recommit to a practice of daily habits, the simple things we do each day that add up to a state of higher health. For us, these include our minimum intake of water, meditation, journaling, a workout, our supplements and even flossing. To ensure consistency with these and any other habits you take on, make a simple chart. List the habits in a single column on the left, and the days of the month across the top. Simply check off each task when you complete it. Watch the page fill up, and know that there's power in repetition. You got this.

RELEASE YOURSELF

One of our favorite Kundalini kriyas, or meditations, for this time of year is the aggressive sounding Fists of Anger. But don't be put off by its name. Fists of Anger is one of the most powerful tools we know for releasing negativity and shifting our mindsets. By removing anger from your field, you open yourself up to grace. And, even if you don't think you have any anger, rest assured, we all do. And, by moving it through the body you open yourself up to its power and can use it to your benefit. Plus, it delivers toned arms and a strong core, all while revealing your most ethereal self. Find grace and beauty in your anger.

HOW TO DO IT: Sit in easy pose or in a seated position on the floor or in a chair. Touch each thumb to the fleshy mounds at the base of the pinkie. Wrap your fingers over your thumb and make a fist. Bring your arms overhead with relaxed, slightly bent elbows. Close your eyes, and begin a version of Breath of Fire through the mouth, with rapid, forceful and even breaths in and out. Then, start moving the arms in a backstroke, alternating arms and coordinating with your rapid breath. Continue for 3 minutes, focusing on the third eye. When the timer goes off, take a deep inhale, hold your breath, interlace your fingers with the palms facing up and your arms extended over your head. Hold your breath, and imagine yourself immersed in white light. Take two more deep breaths in this same posture, release your hands like a cork popping while you forcefully exhale. Allow your hands to slowly lower until they reach the ground. Finish with a long Sat and a short Nam. Repeat daily. Kundalini teaches the power of 40 days. Stick with it, and experience the shift.

PERFORM:
Once daily

WHAT YOU'LL NEED:
Comfortable clothes and a comfortable chair or space on the floor

DURATION:
3 minutes

KERRILYNN'S MORNING MAGIC

Autumn mornings set our intentions and pave the way for productive days. By using this time to ground down, connect to our loved ones and set projects into motion, we activate our most lofty intentions and set ourselves up for productive and prosperous days.

Here's how Kerrilynn begins her day:

"I wake up and head to my favorite chair for 22 minutes of transcendental meditation. I use the app Insight Timer and love to wrap things up by using their feature that allows me to thank others who are meditating with the app as well. There's so much power in connecting to a community of like-minded souls. After meditation, it's time for a tonic. My husband, John, and I start and end each day by talking over a cup (or three!) of adaptogenic herbs. In autumn, we favor herbs that enhance focus and creativity. *Mucuna pruriens*, Rhodiola and Pine Pollen all make the cut. We blend them into a chai tea with coconut butter and tocotrienols and top our drinks with energizing bee pollen. This is sacred time with John and our rescue dogs, Beba and Ricky. Kundalini yoga comes next, and I often have a series of kriyas that I practice in 40-day intervals. I'm especially loving Sudarshan Chakra, which is all about making dreams come true. We take the dogs to Prospect Park, and, if time permits, when we get back home, I start some prep for the evening's dinner. Cutting up cauliflower and onions for an evening soup ensures a healthy and simple meal at day's end. I may squeeze in a face mask, and then it's off to the office for a full day at CAP Beauty.

MOVEMENT FOR IMMUNITY

"Keep up, and you'll be kept up." These wise words from Yogi Bhajan, who brought Kundalini to the West in the 1970s, strike a chord with us this time of year. With the seasonal shift, a return to longer workdays and the back-to-school onset of germs, our immune systems can become compromised. We believe that a daily practice of sweating keeps illness at bay and prevents stagnation from building in our bodies. When we keep it moving, literally and figuratively, we activate and support the immune system, discourage the growth of bacteria and reduce cortisol levels. Here are some key moves to get your body moving. Fit them into your morning or evening routine. No gym required.

VIGOROUS CAT COW. You may be familiar with this stretching series that makes its appearance at the start of almost every yoga class. In this amped-up version, part asana, part pranayama, we go through the same arching and convexing motion, but at a much faster pace than you may be used to.

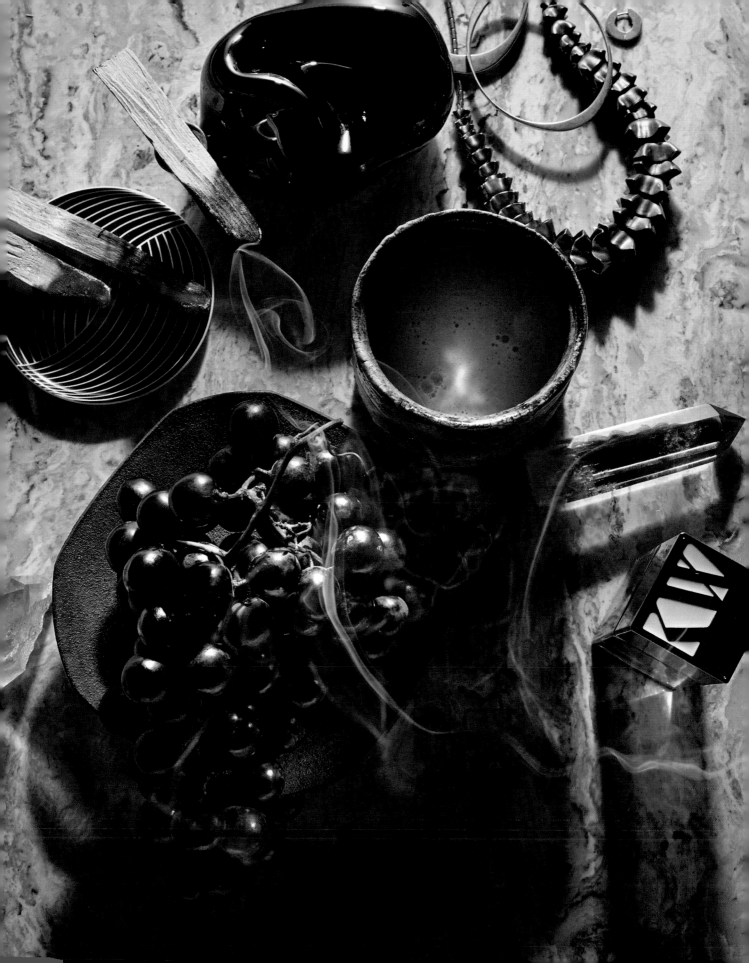

Begin on your hands and knees, with a neutral spine and the tops of your feet touching the floor. Gently lower your back, lift your head and look to the sky as you inhale. This is Cow position. Next, bring your body into Cat position by bringing your belly button toward your spine and rounding your back upward. Your head will drop between your arms as you exhale. Repeat a few times slowly, then pick up the pace, exaggerating the breath as you increase the vigor and speed of your repetitions. Go fast. Let your hair be wild, and get into it. You'll feel the heat build in your body, and you may feel disoriented. Know that you'll come back to neutral soon. Try and build up to a 3-minute practice. Recover in Child's Pose when you're done.

REBOUNDING. All hail the mini trampoline. This playful form of exercise is a staple among the wellness set for its incredible list of benefits, in particular its ability to jumpstart detoxification by boosting lymphatic drainage. A good rebounder can be an investment, and the better models may be easier on the joints, but cheaper versions are also available. We like models from JumpSport and Bellicon. Do your research, then bounce it out.

A little goes a long way. Start with 15 minutes a day (with or without shoes). This can be broken up into shorter sessions. Feet can stay in contact with the trampoline or you can bounce higher for a more advanced practice. Mix it up by trying some alternate moves, tiny jumping jacks, high knee to chest, easy twists. Pair it with Netflix, or put on a great playlist, and get moving.

And, lest you think rebounding is just for hippies and detox junkies like us, you might want to read what NASA has to say. The study is significant, but most notably, their data revealed that rebounding is up to 68-percent more effective than running (rebound-air.com/nasa). We like that it increases bone mass, takes down cellulite, improves digestion and oxygenates the body. Boosted circulation also delivers radiant skin. Such a small investment for such great returns. Shake it up to shake it out.

DANCING. Turn it up, and turn it on. Even a short dance session at home can shift your day and elevate your immune system. Make a playlist (or find one), and get moving. Your physical body will thank you. And, so will your mind. And, with all that home practice, imagine your skills at the next wedding.

STAIR-CLIMBING. There's stairs everywhere, so take advantage of them. Make it a habit to incorporate stair-climbing into your routine. Taking the stairs is a fast-and-effective way to improved health, so get higher and climb your way to happiness. If it worked for Rocky, it'll work for you.

FUTURE TRIPPING (THE RIGHT WAY)

We're dreamers. And, planners. Spending time envisioning your ideal day, week or life is time well spent. It's even better spent when visions become plans and the wheels are set in motion. Allowing ourselves to daydream can be powerful on its own. So often, we are simply working off of today's to-do list, focused on immediate goals and running at top speed. Taking the time to visualize a perfect future can shed light on important values and help us see the big picture. Sometimes, this macro view can overwhelm us, causing us to retreat and dive back into the daily grind. But, stick with it, find delight in the big picture and let it inspire you. Then, back it up with an agile plan. You may find yourself with new priorities, a new outlook and a whole new to-do list.

Be careful to avoid a state of mind that only allows for happiness in a future scenario. This is sometimes referred to as future tripping, and it's not the kind that we're encouraging. You may recognize this as "I'll be happy when I get the promotion, when I lose 5 pounds, when I attain spiritual enlightenment." Be happy now, but indulge your dreams and get planning.

HOW TO DO IT: Sit in a comfortable chair or on the floor in Easy pose. Invite white light in through the crown of your head and allow it to fill your body, feeling hopeful and excited for what's to come. Envision the light moving through you to the core of the Earth, creating a connection to Mother Nature. Allow the light to travel back up though your body, through the crown of your head. Here lies your connection to Source. Then, bask in your perfect future. Where do you live? Who do you love? How does it feel? Get as detailed as you can. You're the architect of all you want.

When you emerge from this blissful meditation, get out your journal, and, without overthinking it, write. You want to integrate this vision into your reality. What did you learn? What surprised you? What aspects of your life are in line with, or at odds with, your dreams?

After a few minutes of freestyle writing, it's time to get practical. This is where dreams become reality. After all, and in the words of French poet Antoine de Saint-Exupéry, "A goal without a plan is just a wish."

DIVIDE YOUR LIFE INTO CATEGORIES THAT ARE RELEVANT TO YOUR GOALS. SOME WE LIKE ARE: health and fitness, career, friends and family, romantic love, finances, spirituality, art and objects, self-development, philanthropy and home. Then, create broad pictures for each of them. These could be in list form or a more narrative version. It's up to you. These goals won't happen overnight, but what can you do today, this week or this month to get closer? Print out calendars and get specific. We've said it before, but it's worth repeating: Enjoy the process, and future trip the right way.

PERFORM:
As needed

WHAT YOU'LL NEED:
A comfortable seat, a journal and calendar pages

DURATION:
1 to 2 hours

A MEDITATION PRACTICE

PERFORM: One or two times daily

WHAT YOU'LL NEED: A comfortable seat, pillow or space on the floor

DURATION: 3 to 22 minutes

Revolution begins within. And, a quiet mind is the catalyst for true change. Seemingly, nothing is simpler than sitting still, yet a meditation practice can elude even the most well-intentioned of us. We overthink it. We get restless. Its benefits are not always obvious. And, worst of all, we judge ourselves for our inability to clear our thoughts. But, upon learning that all of this is part of the process, even for the most experienced practitioner, we look at meditation in a new light, embrace the imperfections and finally commit. The practice is in the practice.

There are countless styles of meditation and ways to practice, some still, some active. Find one that is right for you, and dedicate yourself. With nutrition and fitness, we encourage diversity, but in the case of meditation, we see real value in choosing a style, and calling it our own. It's so easy to jump between practices, especially when we don't see results, but the power here is in consistency. Let yourself go deep, and see what happens over time.

According to Robin Berzin, MD, founder of Parsley Health in New York City, meditation is the single most important thing we can do for our health. When she shared this at CAP Beauty, Cindy asked hopefully if Savasana counts? Wishful thinking. So many of us like to cite flow activities like cooking, yoga, running or reading as forms of meditation. While any activity that encourages a state of flow is fantastic, it's not the same as sitting quietly. This is where you'll reap meditation's true benefits: the physical, mental and spiritual. And, the benefits are vast. Meditation increases the gray matter in our brains, lowers cortisol, increases focus, reduces blood pressure, alleviates anxiety, tackles depression and insomnia and puts the body in a state of heightened healing. Given this list, it's shocking that so many of us resist this simple practice.

Here are some of our practices. Spend a few weeks testing them out, then choose one that resonates. Feel free to do more than one. Kerrilynn practices both transcendental meditation (TM) and Kundalini, and finds them to complement each other. And, adding in a special event like a large-group meditation or sound bath is always powerful.

TRANSCENDENTAL MEDITATION. TM, a form of Vedic meditation, was made famous by the Beatles, who studied under master teacher Maharishi Mahesh Yogi. Vedic traditions rely on the repetition of a simple mantra to focus the mind, crowding out thoughts and easing the body into a state of deep rest. TM and other forms of Vedic meditation are formally learned through a certified teacher who stays with you for life. We were lucky enough to study with Bob Roth, the executive director of the David Lynch Foundation in New York City, and he changed our lives. Find your teacher, and change yours.

KUNDALINI. Yogi Bhajan brought Kundalini, also known as Householder's yoga, to us. It's called Householder's yoga because it can be practiced anywhere and is available to all. The science of Kundalini incorporates breath, movement and focus into short (or long) routines called kriyas. These kriyas raise your Kundalini or Life Force Energy, something we all have in varying states. Wake up and raise this energy to reach spiritual enlightenment. Moreover, each kriya targets a specific goal or intention. Attract prosperity, increase magnetism, raise your sexual energy or encourage youthfulness and beauty. Kundalini kriyas are an active form of meditation, appealing to those who have a harder time sitting. This ancient practice has modern appeal. Find a Kundalini center or learn the kriyas through short videos online. We love RA MA TV (rama-tv.com). Sat Nam.

LOVING KINDNESS. In this beautiful Buddhist practice, we shower others and ourselves with love and gratitude. Also known as metta, this simple-yet-profound technique crowds out negativity and elevates our state of mind. It has been found to increase empathy and relieve depression. Begin by repeating the phrase "May I be happy." Then, direct this wish toward someone you love or someone you feel grateful for. Next, direct it toward someone you feel neutral toward, and then direct it toward someone who is presenting a challenge. Finally, offer this phrase up to the universe: "May all beings everywhere be happy." You can make the practice your own. Try "May I be healthy and strong. May I be filled with ease. May I be surrounded with love." This is also a great practice to begin with kids or practice with a partner. This practice has become one of the favorite times of the day for Cindy's daughter, Sally. Be love. And, start them young.

CRYSTALS FOR MANIFESTING

These are the stones we keep on hand to call in what we desire and to attract and create abundance. Dream big, then ground down to fly high.

AMETHYST: Illuminate your path with this lilac beauty. Clarify and connect to your higher goals.

PEARL: Keep the faith. This vital component of manifesting is strengthened through the presence of pearl.

GARNET: The stone of health encourages a state of body and state of mind ripe for attraction.

FLUORITE: This supernatural stone allows for higher levels of communication. Ask the universe. Receive.

HOWLITE: Encourage a state of strength and calm when asking for what you desire. A tranquil sea is a powerful sea.

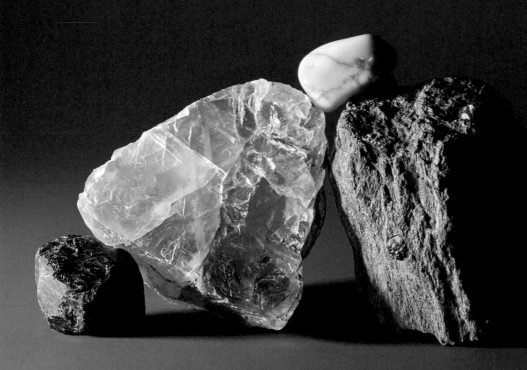

MASTERMINDING

We are as good as the people who surround us. So, to reach our highest state, we make a conscious choice to align ourselves with the best and the brightest. Mastermind groups are a staple of classic entrepreneurial culture. Coined by Napoleon Hill, author of the seminal *Think and Grow Rich*, masterminding is the practice of formally and consistently meeting with a group of peers, usually fellow entrepreneurs or other creators, to share insights and resources, critique one another's work and offer encouragement and support. Expanding your network is an obvious benefit as well.

The idea and inception of CAP Beauty actually sprang from a weekly mastermind meeting. Kerrilynn shared her dream for a natural beauty store, and Cindy encouraged her to pursue this, without letting it die. When they decided to partner, the wheels were set in motion. Even though they had never formally worked together, years of masterminding gave them insight into each other's working styles and ethics, paving the way for a perfect partnership. Whether or not a new company forms from your group, there's much to gain, and there's power in the practice. Most important, this is a safe space, a place to offer and receive thoughtful and sometimes challenging feedback and a place to learn about your own habits and what works best for others. Support others in their highest ambitions and know that they support yours. Grow together.

HOW TO DO IT: Think of people whose work and mission you admire. Do you have something to offer to them and they to you? Select your group carefully and with intention. The plan is to stay together for the long haul. Groups may be as few as three or as many as eight. Small worked well for us. Decide on a day and set it in your calendar as a non-negotiable commitment. It's no surprise again here that consistency is key.

Pick a place where you can spend some time, that is convenient to all and preferably has healthy food and drinks. Set up a schedule for the meeting and determine how long each member will hold court. We found that 15 minutes per member worked well. For larger groups, you may try alternating weeks. Stay on task, and use a timer. It's easy to get sidetracked, but discipline is vital. If these are people you want to talk with personally, make a date for dinner or stay after and chat. Keep it business. One person takes notes and circulates them after each meeting. This creates continuity between meetings. Begin each meeting with an invocation you write together. Why are you here? What do you want to manifest? How can you serve? Then, dive right into each 15-minute block. Serve yourself by serving others.

AUTUMN ENERGY CLEARING

PERFORM: One or two times daily

WHAT YOU'LL NEED: Palo Santo, matches, and a fireproof dish

DURATION: 5 to 10 minutes

Channel your inner shaman. The act of burning, also known as smudging, has been performed for centuries by healers across the globe. Thought to promote positive energy, smudging dissolves negativity through the intentional act of burning a natural and fragrant substance. While other substances may be used, this season we choose Palo Santo, also known as holy wood, for its grounding and earthy scent. Watch the smoke rise and dissipate and know that positive thoughts and prayers rise with the smoke to be met by Source energy. Embrace the beautiful scent of the wood, and enjoy taking this time to honor and reclaim your space. Love yourself by caring for your environment. Beauty is all around.

HOW TO DO IT: Find a comfortable spot in a favorite area of your home, and sit. Hold the Palo Santo in your hands and take three deep cleansing breaths, connecting to yourself and the wood. Let go of all your worries from the day, knowing that this ritual removes concerns and gives way to light. Call upon your higher power, be that God, Mother Earth, a spirit guide or Source, whatever you connect with. Ask for help in clearing your space and filling it with the energies of love. Light the Palo Santo at one end. If the flame does not dissipate on its own gently snuff it out, so the wood smolders. Visit all corners of your space with the Palo Santo, while repeating a simple mantra. We like "Let there be love, let there be light." Once you've treated every area of your space, lay the wood in a fireproof dish (we like Fornasetti!) and allow it to continue smoking safely. Breathe deeply and give thanks for your space and the positive energies it now holds.

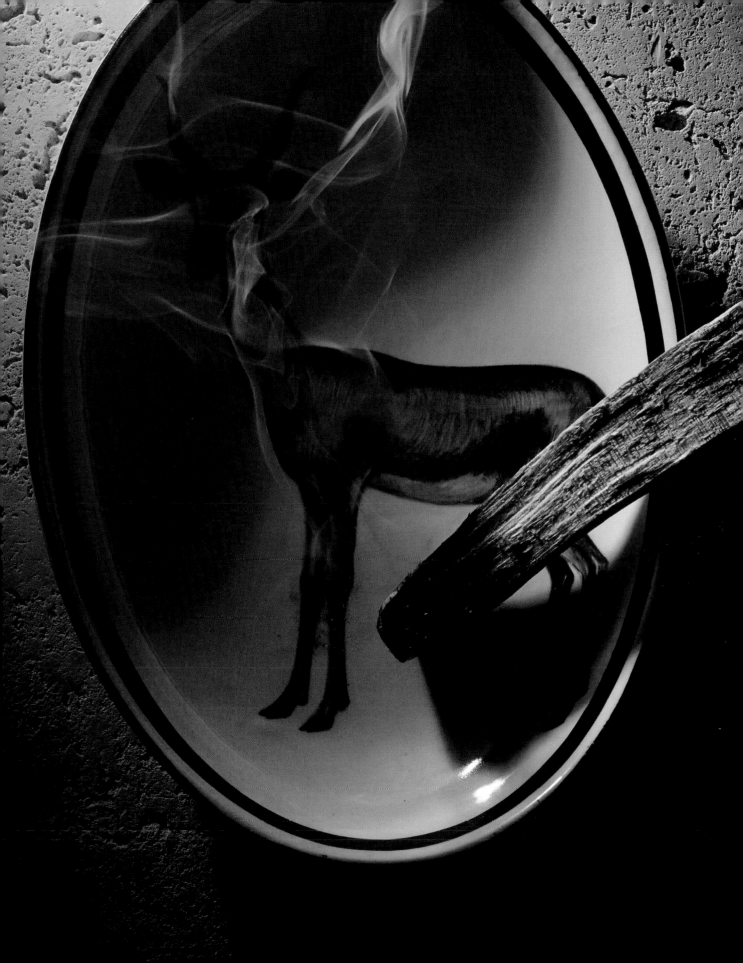

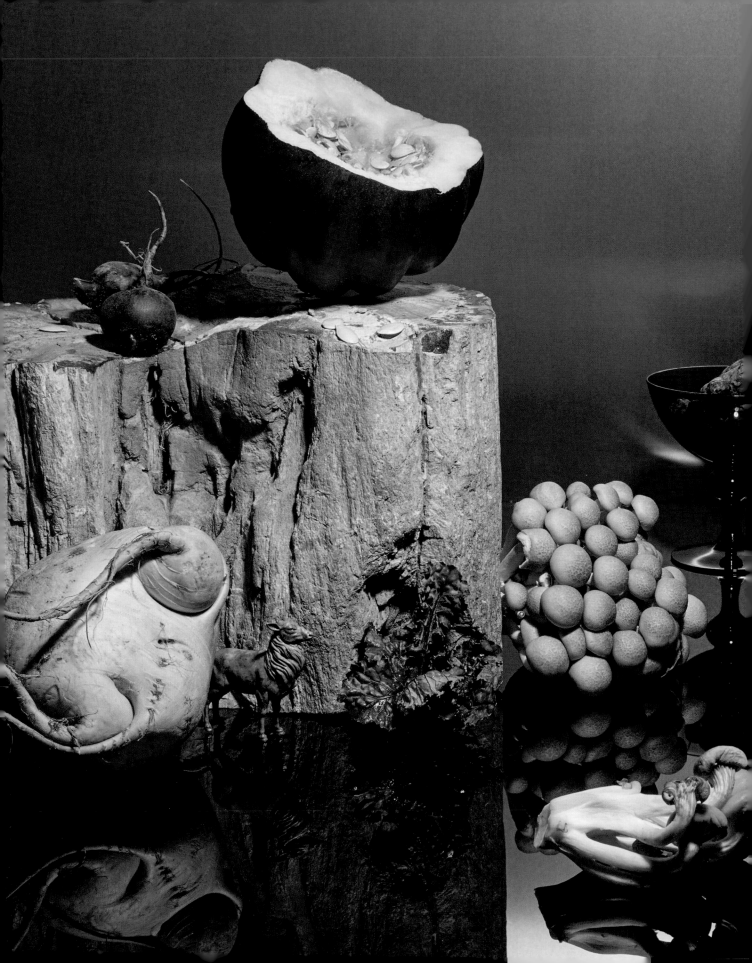

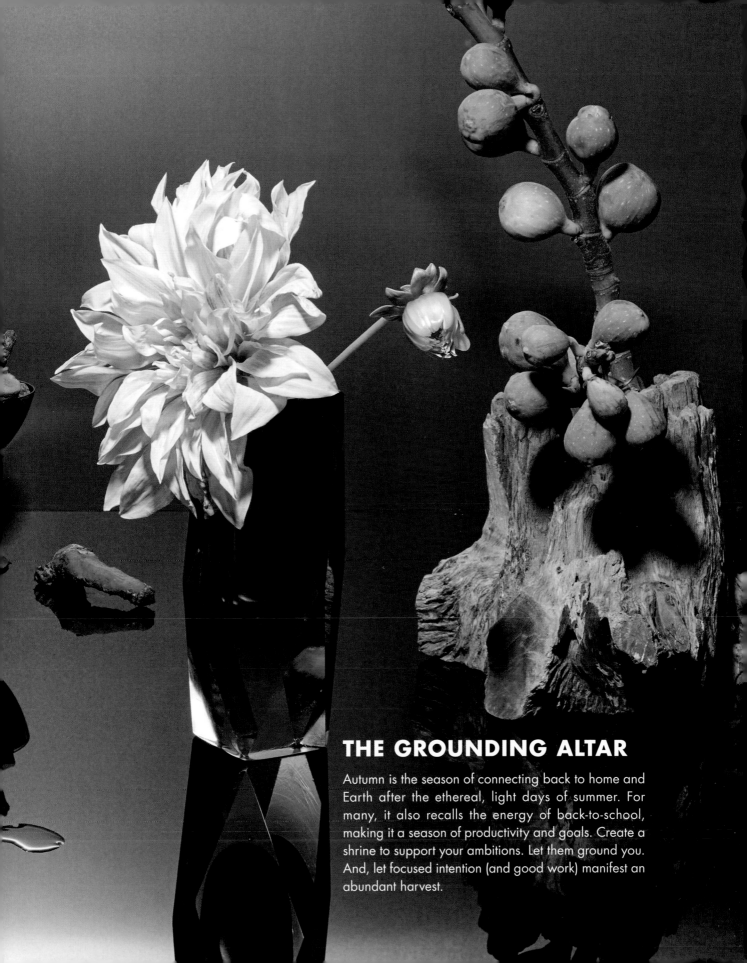

THE GROUNDING ALTAR

Autumn is the season of connecting back to home and Earth after the ethereal, light days of summer. For many, it also recalls the energy of back-to-school, making it a season of productivity and goals. Create a shrine to support your ambitions. Let them ground you. And, let focused intention (and good work) manifest an abundant harvest.

CLOSET CLEARING

PERFORM:
Twice a year,
or as needed

WHAT YOU'LL NEED:
A patient and honest
friend, a note pad
and a camera

DURATION:
4 to 6 hours

Refine, reset, renew. As with all things, we believe in the power of creating space. Of only keeping things in your life that create true happiness and ease. We also love a great outfit. When your closet overwhelms you, when it's packed to the brim but you have nothing to wear, the best defense is to dive deep, isolate what you love and toss the rest. Cindy did this project with a close friend years ago, and it was a transformative act. For her and her friend. Your mornings (and your loved ones) will thank you.

HOW TO DO IT: Invite a trusted and stylish friend to help. Make sure that he or she understands that they may be engaged for a full afternoon. Have snacks on hand and a favorite drink. Then, get to work. Start with separates; pants and skirts are good. Try on each pair and judge it on its real merit, not its history, its maker or its cost. Then, ask yourself and your friend if they flatter you. Do you feel good? Are they past their prime, stained or threadbare? Be honest and ruthless, and keep emotions at bay. If they pass the test, your friend can jot them down on a master list. Otherwise, make a bag for donations or recycling. Systematically go through all bottoms, then all tops, and then go through the same process with dresses. Finally, take a survey of accessories. Lay out belts, shoes, and so on.

Once you've created a list of separates, start building complete looks and ask yourself what each outfit needs. More often than not, it's already in your closet, but you may discover a few key pieces that are missing. Add them to your list, and shopping will become intentional and purposeful. And, when the exercise is done, you'll have your own personal style guide and a lot more space in your closet.

As you try everything on, ask your friend to take notes and list each perfect outfit you discover. You can even make a spreadsheet with each look, and you can cross reference it when packing for a trip. Locate each outfit built around the same skirt or shoes. Packing will be simplified. Put in the time now to free up time later, and leave morning stress behind. You might even start getting to work early.

THE SYSTEMS CALENDAR

Take note! We've found that assigning certain days of the week to certain tasks ensures that it all gets done and clears our minds of to-do-list chatter. As David Allen, author of *Getting Things Done*, says, "The mind is for having ideas, not holding them." Fix it and forget it, and open yourself up to spontaneity. This tip has massively impacted Kerrilynn's life and allows for more freedom during the week, knowing what each day brings.

HOW TO DO IT: Write out all of your tasks for the week, including some self care rituals. We're talking laundry, gardening, paying bills, grocery shopping, cleaning the house, you get the idea. Then, create a digital homekeeping calendar, and assign each item as a recurring event. We like to do errands on Wednesdays, cook for the week on Sunday mornings, take a bath on Thursday nights. Plan as best you can, but edit the calendar as you need. And, enjoy the peace of mind of knowing that it will all get done.

EXTRA CREDIT: For more in-depth projects, like cleaning out the medicine chest and washing area rugs, we turn to our homekeeping hero, flylady (flylady.net), and her ingenious method of creating an area of focus for each week. When the kitchen is the focus, you may spend 15 minutes one morning wiping down the fridge and 15 minutes the next day on the silverware drawer. Planning these short, effective and constantly rotating tasks has revolutionized the way that we keep house. More often than not, we don't have 2 hours, but we can find 15 minutes a day. As always, consistency rules. Learn to love your space.

THE RECIPES:

HARVEST MOON

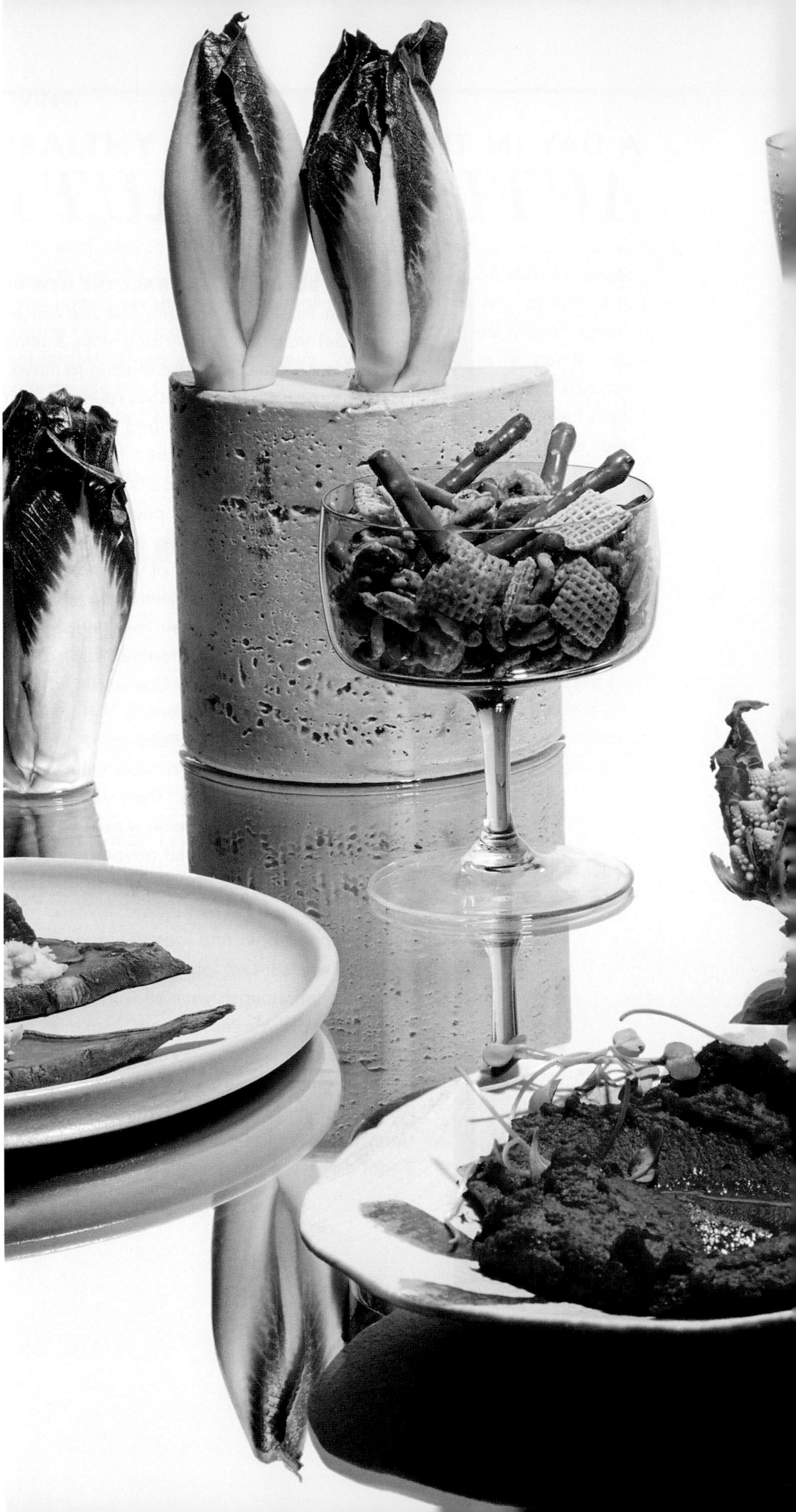

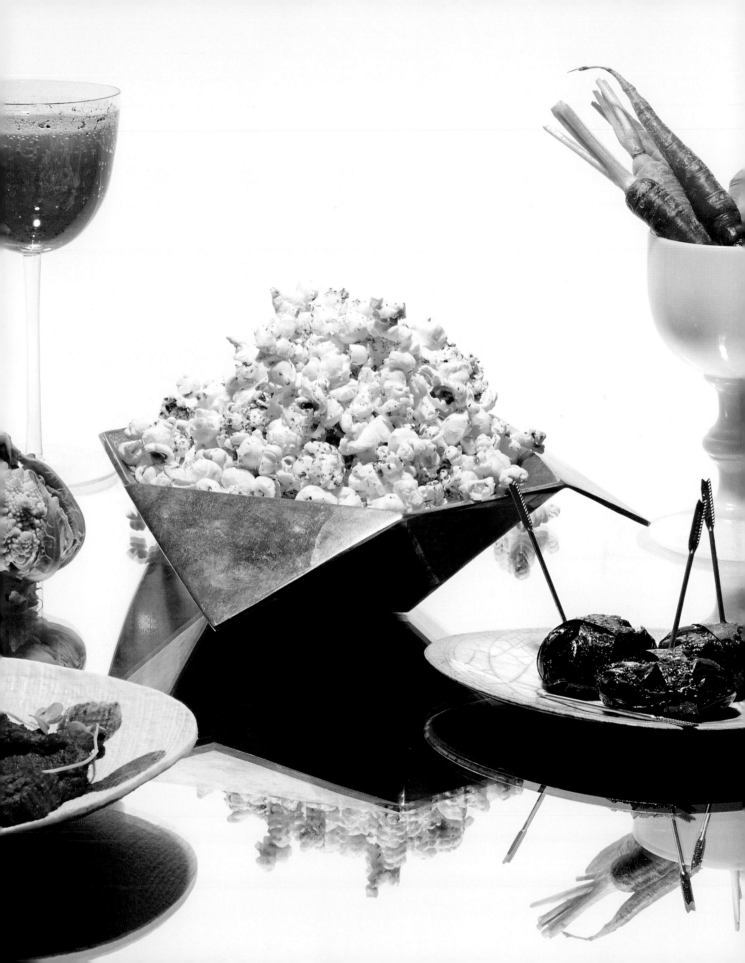

THE NEW WAVE OPEN HOUSE

Getting friends together is a rite of autumn. We love to reunite with loved ones after a busy summer, and a casual open house by day or night with delicious snacks and drinks invites friends to come and go, reconnect and dig in. We reinterpret party snacks to leave everyone feeling better and brighter. Even the drinks pack a superfood punch. Imbibe in joy, and get the party started.

HERE'S HOW TO DO IT: Prepare a scattering of High Vibrational party food and set up stations of snacks throughout the house. Something by the fire, something by the bar. Things will flow. Set a separate table, later in the day or evening with sweeter fare alongside teas or toddies. At an open house, the idea is for friends to come and go, but we like it when they stick around. Keep friends close by keeping them fed.

SAVORY SNACKS

Smoked Sevilla Popcorn (page 65)

Kyoto Krunch (page 63)

Reimagined Party Mix (opposite)

Angels on Horseback (below)

Magenta Miso Smash (page 173)

Source Soup (page 227)

Beachy Beet Chips (page 239)

Assorted autumn crudités

Sweet Potato Toasts (opposite)

DESSERT BUFFET

This Little Figgy Crumb Pudding (page 162)

Pumpkin Pie Pudding (page 181)

Chocolate Apex Cookies (page 180)

COCKTAILS

Pine Pollen Fizz (page 130)

Elderflower Champagne Cocktail (page 160)

Sea Buckthorn Spike (page 160)

ANGELS ON HORSEBACK

2 tablespoons olive oil

12 almonds

Himalayan pink salt, to taste

Black pepper

12 dates, pitted

2 toasted nori sheets, cut into 1-inch by 6-inch strips

Preheat the oven to 350°F. Pour the oil over the almonds and season with a little salt and pepper. Stuff each date with an almond and roast for 5 to 10 minutes. Remove from oven, wrap with a nori sheet and close with a toothpick. Add more salt, if needed.

MAKES 12

REIMAGINED PARTY MIX

½ cup coconut oil

2 tablespoons Sea Clear or miso

1½ tablespoons Berbere (page 267)

1 tablespoon Worcestershire sauce

1 cup gluten-free pretzels

1 cup Roasted Chickpea Croutons (page 41)

1 cup tamari almonds

1½ cups Chex corn cereal

1½ cups Chex rice cereal

2 cups puffed brown rice

Preheat the oven to 250°F. Add the oil to a large saucepan and mix in the Sea Clear or miso, berbere and Worcestershire sauce and melt on stovetop. Set aside. Toss the pretzels, spicy chickpeas, almonds, corn Chex, rice Chex and puffed brown rice in the largest bowl you have, and coat to cover with the coconut oil mixture. Make sure to mix this really well, then turn it out onto a baking sheet. Bake for 25 minutes, shaking and turning from time to time. When slightly browned, remove from oven and enjoy. It's party time!

SERVES MANY

SWEET POTATO TOASTS

2 sweet potatoes

Cashew Quark (page 253)

Berbere (page 267)

Relish the Relish (page 259; optional)

Slice the sweet potatoes into ¼-inch to ½-inch slices using a mandoline. Place them in a toaster oven or under a broiler and toast for about 5 minutes. You want to get them pretty toasted, so however many times you need to toast them, do it. If broiling, be sure to flip them over and watch them closely. Once toasted, top with the Cashew Quark, berbere and relish. Enjoy!

SERVES 6 TO 8

The Fig Newton got reinvented. And, it's better than ever. We took everything we love about the classic cookie and reinterpreted it into another love of ours, the upside-down cake. Jammy on the top, and sweet on the bottom, this little figgy is coming home.

THIS LITTLE FIGGY CRUMB PUDDING

½ cup coconut oil, plus more for greasing the pan

8 to 10 fresh figs, halved

1 cup coconut flour

1 teaspoon baking powder

1 teaspoon cinnamon

½ teaspoon Himalayan pink salt

½ cup Aquafaba (page 261)

½ cup coconut sugar

1 teaspoon vanilla extract or ½ vanilla bean

Preheat the oven to 350°F. Place a piece of parchment paper on the bottom of a 9" springform pan. Grease both the parchment and the sides of the pan with the reserved coconut oil. Place the figs, cut-side down, on the bottom of the pan and set aside.

In a medium mixing bowl, whisk together the flour, baking powder, cinnamon and salt.

Place the aquafaba and sugar in the bowl of a mixer. Whip on high speed until stiff peaks form. Add in the vanilla and coconut oil and whip for 2 additional minutes. Working in stages, add in the flour mixture until just combined. Pour the batter over the figs. Place the pan on a baking sheet to prevent any spills and bake for 20 to 30 minutes, until a knife inserted in the middle comes out clean. Allow to cool. Remove from the pan and gently flip, using a serving plate to assist you.

SERVES 6 TO 8

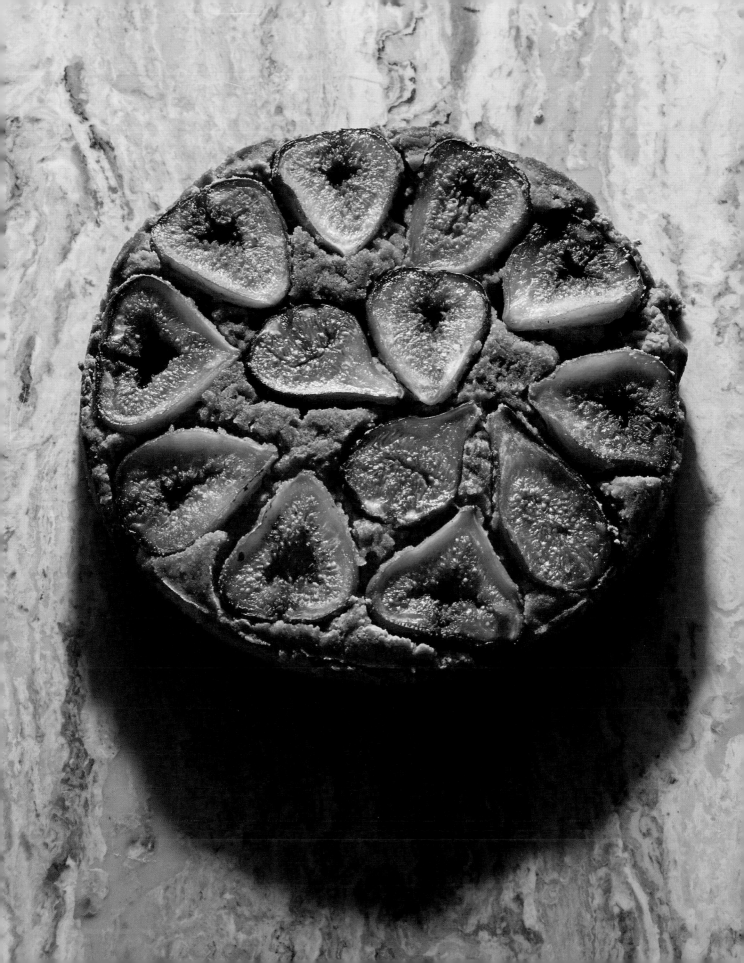

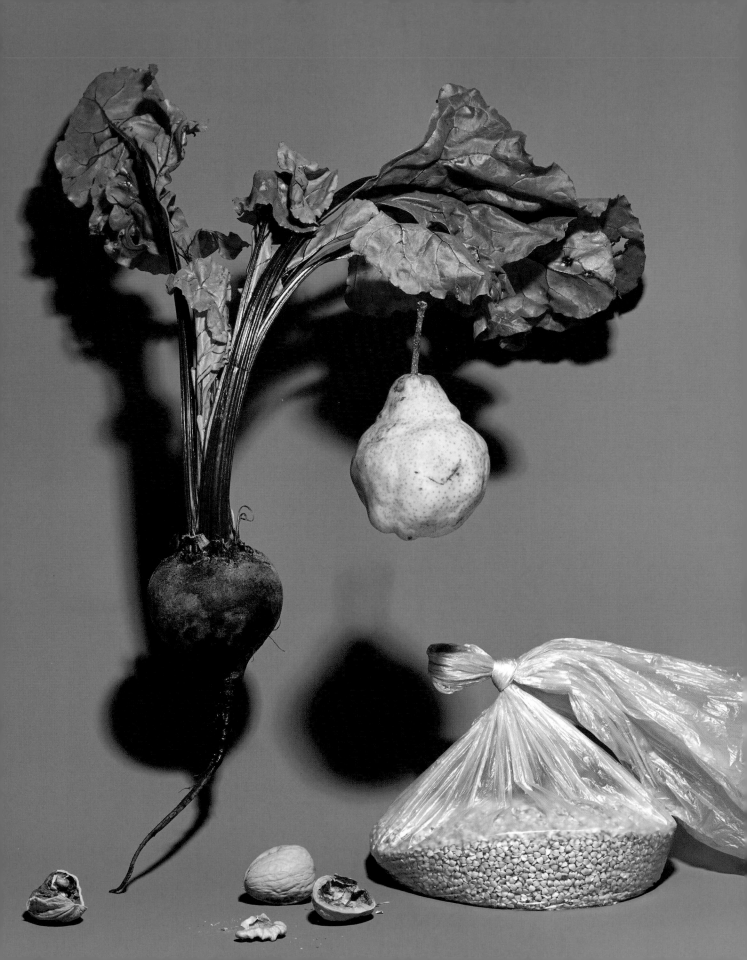

Buckwheat imparts an earthy, nutty flavor that offsets the sweet additions to this breakfast bowl. A pseudo-grain like quinoa, it's higher in protein and easier to digest than other grains. A perfect start to an autumn morning.

MOSCOW MORNING PORRIDGE

1 cup buckwheat groats

4 dates, pitted and chopped

2½ cups filtered water

1 small beet, peeled and grated

1 ripe pear, chopped

1 cinnamon stick

1 tablespoon grated ginger

¼ teaspoon Himalayan pink salt

2 tablespoons coconut butter

Toasted walnuts

Bee pollen

Honey or maple syrup

In a medium bowl, soak the groats and dates in water overnight. Strain, rinse and transfer to a medium saucepan. Add the 2½ cups water, beet, pear, cinnamon, ginger and salt. Bring to a boil over medium heat, then reduce to a simmer. Cook until most of the liquid has been absorbed, 10 to 15 minutes. Remove from the heat and stir in the coconut butter. Top with the walnuts, bee pollen, and honey or syrup.

SERVES 4

BUCKWHEAT GROATS

This little seed packs a punch. While many of us think of buckwheat as a grain, it's actually a fruit seed that is closely related to one of our favorite spring fruits: rhubarb. A perfect substitute for traditional cereals, buckwheat groats uplevel your morning oatmeal. High in magnesium, which has been known to relax blood vessels, buckwheat contributes to a healthy cardiovascular system and strong circulation.

Cooked grapes add a winey and caramelized richness to any dish they grace and pair perfectly with dark bitter greens. They're classically added to the pan with roast chicken or sausage. Our version substitutes prebiotic-rich Jerusalem artichokes, creating a bitter, sweet and earthy meal to celebrate the season.

BITTERSWEET ROAST

1 large bunch purple grapes

1 red onion, sliced into thick half-moons

1 pound Jerusalem artichokes, washed

Splash of olive oil

Himalayan pink salt

Black pepper

2 big bunches of broccoli rabe or other bitter greens, cleaned and trimmed

Preheat the oven to 350°F. Wash the grapes, remove them from the vine and add them to the bottom of a roasting dish (we love a French porcelain baker for this). Add the onion, whole artichokes, oil and a generous amount of salt and pepper, to taste. Then toss to coat everything. Bake for 25 to 30 minutes, tossing once halfway through. You will know the dish is ready when a knife can be easily inserted in the Jerusalem artichokes and the grapes are caramelized.

About 5 minutes before the artichokes are ready, steam the greens in a steamer pot. Place them on a platter and top with the roasted grapes and artichokes, allowing the cooking juices to dress the greens.

SERVES 2 TO 4

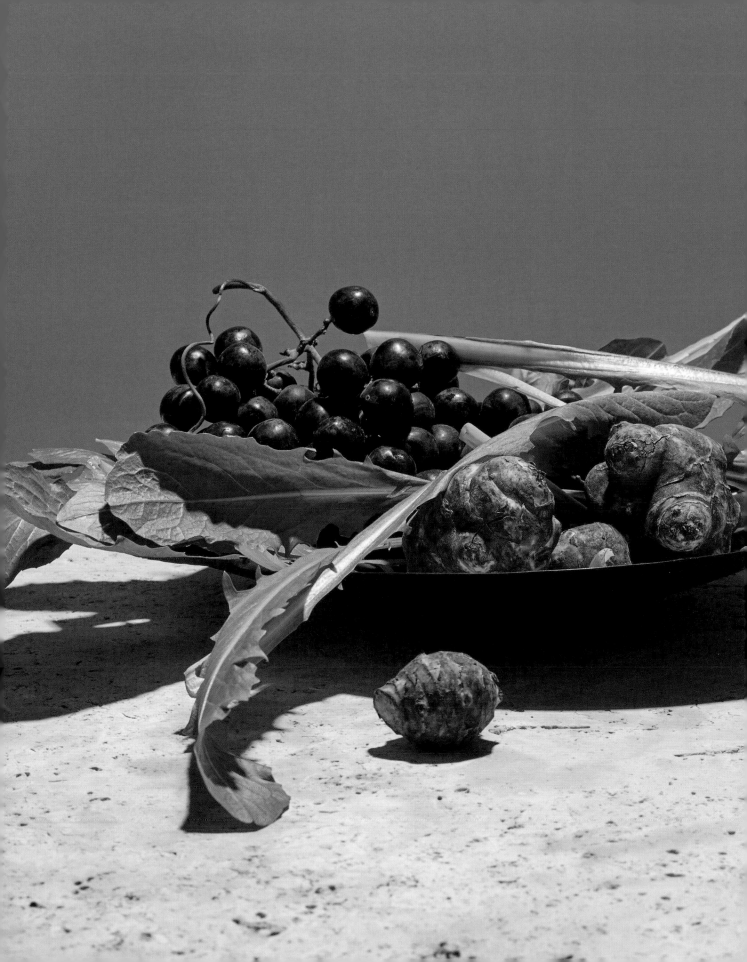

Raw beets married with oranges, coconut, avocado and fennel put a fresh and unexpected spin on the bounties of autumn. This simple-yet-elegant meal is the perfect starter for your next dinner party.

BEET CEVICHE

2 medium beets, scrubbed

½ shallot, minced

Juice and zest of 1 orange

1 teaspoon ume plum vinegar

½ cup coconut water

¼ teaspoon Himalayan pink salt

1 fennel bulb, sliced ⅛-inch

Olive oil, for drizzling

Orange segments

Avocado slices

Toasted hazelnuts

Using a mandoline, slice the beets ⅛ inch thick. Arrange them in a deep storage container. Mix the shallot, orange juice and zest, vinegar, coconut water and salt together in a small bowl and then pour on top of the beets. Refrigerate overnight. Remove the beets from the soaking liquid and arrange them on a platter. Drizzle some oil over the top and then add the fennel, oranges, avocado and nuts. You can use the leftover marinade as a dressing for this or other salad dishes.

SERVES 4

Sassy and aggressive, puttanesca is one of Kerrilynn's favorite pasta sauces. She introduced it to her family years ago on a ski trip (the perfect aprés-ski meal), and it's still in their weekly rotation. Rumored to be inspired by "The Ladies of the Night," this sultry-and-spicy dish has us coming back for more. Paired with zucchini noodles, this lighter take on the traditional dish guarantees room for seconds.

A SAUCE FOR THE NIGHT

3 tablespoons olive oil, plus more for finishing

2 sweet onions, diced

2 heads of garlic, minced

1 red bell pepper, seeded and diced

10 small to medium tomatoes, chopped coarsely, or 2 (28 ounces each) cans of tomatoes

1 tablespoon Himalayan pink salt, plus more if needed

½ tablespoon freshly ground black pepper

12 botija olives, pitted and chopped

8 to 10 capers, minced

1 to 2 chiles de arbol, seeded and minced, or ½ teaspoon crushed red pepper, plus more if needed

4 to 6 zucchini, spiralized

Handful of Italian parsley, chopped finely

Heat a heavy-bottomed pan over medium heat and warm the oil. Add the onions and cook for 8 to 10 minutes, or until translucent. Add the garlic halfway through the cooking time. Add the bell peppers, tomatoes, salt and pepper and cook for another 8 to 10 minutes over high heat. You want the sauce to cook down, so bring it to a low boil. Add in the olives, capers and chiles and continue to simmer for 10 minutes.

Meanwhile, heat the zucchini through in a large skillet over medium heat. Pour the sauce over the zucchini and toss to thoroughly combine. Finish the sauce with more chiles, salt and oil, if desired. Top zucchini with the sauce and sprinkle with the parsley.

SERVES 4

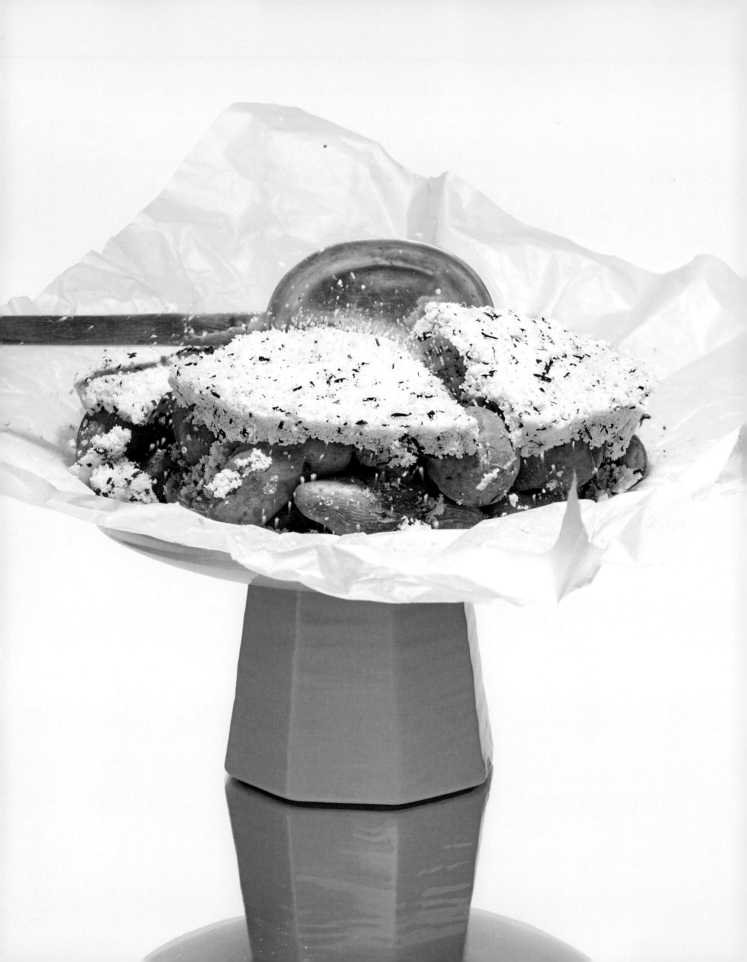

Inspired by the master of minimalism, John Pawson, and his brilliant cookbook *Living and Eating*, these smoky, tea-infused potatoes are an elegant and mysterious plant-based nod to the classic tea-smoked chicken. Perfect for a night in front of the fire, add this exotic dish to your dinner party rotation, and share the power of plants with your closest friends.

PAWSON'S POTATOES

1 pound sea salt (about 4 cups)

⅓ cup Lapsang Souchong tea leaves

Filtered water

1½ to 2 pounds small red or fingerling potatoes

Lentils with Dandelion Greens (below)

Preheat the oven to 400°F.

Place the salt and tea in a large mixing bowl. Add water 1 tablespoon at a time until a consistency like wet sand is achieved. Place one-third of the mixture onto a large parchment-lined baking sheet. Add the potatoes and cover them with the remaining salt mixture. Make sure to cover the potatoes entirely, because you want them to steam inside. Roast for 45 minutes to 1 hour, or until a knife can easily pierce through the potatoes. Remove from the oven and allow to rest for 10 minutes. Crack open the salt crust, remove the potatoes, discard the salt and tea crust and serve them atop Lentils with Dandelion Greens.

SERVES 4 TO 6

LENTILS WITH DANDELION GREENS

2 tablespoons olive or coconut oil

1 onion, diced

4 cloves garlic, minced

2 cups dried French lentils, rinsed

1 teaspoon chili flakes

1 tablespoon Himalayan pink salt, plus more if needed

6 cups filtered water

1 bunch of thyme

2 bay leaves

1 bunch of dandelion greens, chopped

Fresh lemon juice

Heat the oil in a large stockpot. Add the onion and garlic and cook on medium heat until the onion becomes soft and translucent. Add in the lentils, chili flakes and salt. Stir. Add in the water, thyme and bay leaves. Bring to a boil, reduce to a simmer and cook on medium heat until the lentils become tender and most of the liquid has been absorbed, about 20 minutes, but check after 15 minutes to make sure they aren't overcooked. Remove the bay leaves, toss in the dandelion greens and turn off the heat. Season, to taste, with lemon juice and adjust salt, to taste.

SERVES 4 TO 6

Grazie porcini. These dried mushrooms impart more than their share of earthy and rich flavor, making them a perfect pantry staple. This is Italy incarnate, but pairs perfectly with Japanese buckwheat soba for a love child of a meal.

PORCINI LOVE CHILD

¼ cup dried porcini mushrooms

2 cups hot water

1 package buckwheat soba or 100% buckwheat pasta

2 tablespoons olive oil

2 cloves garlic, smashed and chopped

4 cups mixed fresh mushrooms, coarsely chopped

Himalayan pink salt

½ bunch parsley, coarsely chopped

Several big handfuls of baby arugula

Black pepper

½ lemon

Place the porcini in a small mixing bowl and just cover with the water. Let stand until softened. Meanwhile, cook the soba or pasta according to the package directions for al dente. Remove the porcini from the water (reserve the water), and coarsely chop them. In a large sauté pan, heat the oil over medium heat. Add the garlic, and sauté a minute or so, until softened and fragrant. Add the porcini and fresh mushrooms and a large pinch of salt, and sauté until the mushrooms soften. Add the reserved porcini water to the pan and continue cooking until the liquid is reduced to about 1 cup. Strain the pasta, add it to the mushroom sauce and toss to combine. Distribute among four pasta bowls. Top each with a handful of parsley and arugula, more salt, pepper and a squeeze of lemon juice.

SERVES 4

BUCKWHEAT SOBA

We rely heavily on Japan for inspiration and that, of course, extends to our kitchens. Having a pack of nutrient-dense buckwheat noodles in your pantry is the fastest route to a meal inspired by the flavors of one of our favorite countries. Perfect for those of us who crave the satisfaction of a noodle dish without the gluten, these noodles are a rich source of phyto-nutrients and heart-healthy antioxidants and a great source of protein and manganese, encouraging collagen production for beautiful skin. Eat like the Japanese, and welcome the glow.

This magenta dip is delicious with crudités and makes a perfect addition to bowls and salads. With an unexpected dose of miso and coriander's nod to the Middle East, this mashup is UN approved. And, totally delicious.

MAGENTA MISO SMASH

2 medium beets, rinsed

2 tablespoons chickpea miso

1 small clove garlic, chopped

1 teaspoon ground coriander

2 teaspoons lemon juice

2 tablespoons olive oil

1 tablespoon filtered water

Himalayan pink salt

Preheat the oven to 400°F. Wrap the beets up tightly in aluminum foil or parchment paper. Roast for 45 minutes to 1 hour, or until you can pierce through them easily with a knife. Remove from the oven, unwrap and allow to cool. Peel by rubbing the skin away from the beet and chop the beets (you should have about 2 cups).

Add the miso and garlic to a food processor and process until broken down. Add the beets, coriander, lemon juice, oil and water and continue to process until everything comes together in a smooth paste, scraping down the sides as necessary. Season with salt, to taste.

MAKES 2 CUPS

There's nothing like nachos. And, when cravings call, we give in to this High Vibrational interpretation of, quite simply, the best party food there is. Invite your friends, and let it shine. This is nacho average recipe.

NACHO NACHOS

CHIPS

1 small butternut squash, necks only, peeled and halved

2 tablespoons olive oil or coconut oil

Himalayan pink salt

AVOCADO MASH

2 avocados, pitted, halved and scooped

1 tablespoon olive oil

Juice of 1 lime

¼ teaspoon Himalayan pink salt

PICKLED HIBISCUS

¼ cup ume plum vinegar

¼ cup filtered water

½ teaspoon coconut sugar

¼ teaspoon Himalayan pink salt

2 tablespoons dried hibiscus flowers

1 cup Sunflower Queso (page 252)

4 radishes, thinly sliced

½ cup cilantro leaves

2 scallions, white and light green parts only, thinly sliced

Preheat the oven to 375°F. Bring a large pot of water to boil over high heat.

To make the chips: Using a mandoline, slice the squash into half-moons about ⅛ inch thick. In batches, drop them into the boiling water and cook for about 2 minutes, or until soft. Remove with a slotted spatula and transfer to a towel lined plate. Allow to cool. Pat dry with a paper towel, making sure to absorb any excess water. Transfer to a few parchment-lined baking sheets in a single layer with no overlapping. Brush them with the oil and a sprinkle of salt. Bake for 10 minutes. Flip the chips and bake for 5 minutes more. If they look golden brown and a bit crispy, remove them. If not, leave them in for an additional 5 minutes, keeping a close eye on them so they don't burn (some may finish sooner than others, depending on the thickness and size). The chips will continue to crisp up more once they are removed from the oven. Set aside, and allow them to cool. (Alternatively, you can dehydrate them at 125°F for 18 to 24 hours.)

To make the avocado mash: Combine all ingredients in a medium bowl, and gently mash. Cover and refrigerate.

To make the pickled hibiscus: Add all ingredients except the hibiscus flowers to a small saucepan and set over low heat. Gently warm and stir until the salt and sugar dissolve. Turn off the heat and toss in the flowers. Allow to sit for at least 30 minutes. Strain the flowers from the brine (you can save the brine and use as a base for salad dressings), and set aside.

To assemble: Place a layer of squash chips on a large plate. Warm ½ cup of the Sunflower Queso and drizzle on the chips, then top with half the avocado mash. Make another layer with the remaining chips, queso and avocado mash. Top with the flowers, radishes, cilantro and scallions.

SERVES 4

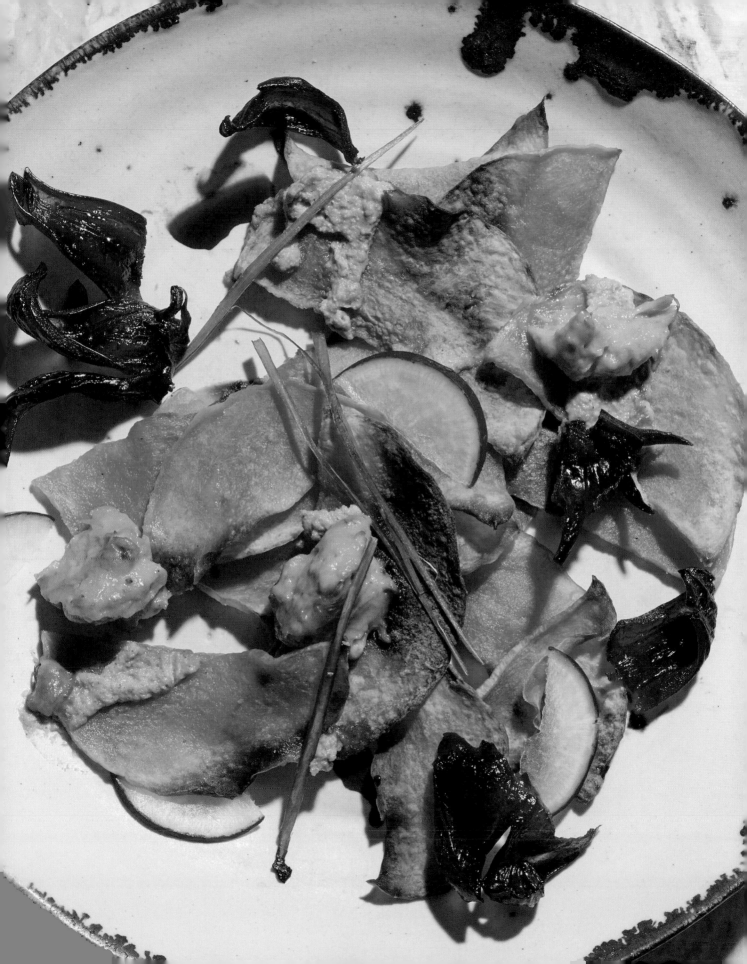

The most stunning colors of the season merge into this taste of early autumn. Frances Boswell, our friend and brilliant acupuncturist, embodies all the beauty of New England and created this love song to the Northeast. Add it to coconut yogurt or buckwheat crepes or serve alongside nut cheeses. A little goes a long way here, so don't be afraid to share. Consider it the perfect end to a day spent at the orchard.

UPSTATE ORCHARD SINK SAUCE

1 bunch Concord grapes

8 apples, peeled, cored and quartered

2 pears, peeled, cored and quartered

2 peaches, peeled, pitted and quartered

8 Italian prune plums, halved, pitted and chopped

½ teaspoon Himalayan pink salt

Remove the grapes from the stems and place them in a small saucepan and cover with about 2 cups of water and bring to a boil over medium heat. Reduce the heat and simmer until the grapes break down, about 4 minutes. Remove from the heat and strain the grapes, collecting the liquid in a large, heavy-bottomed nonreactive pot. Press down on the grapes to extract all the flavor, then discard them. Add the apples, pears, peaches, plums and salt to the pot. Cover and let simmer gently over medium heat just until the fruit breaks down to a nice slightly chunky rustic applesauce consistency, 20 to 30 minutes, though it could take a little longer, depending on ripeness. Remove from the heat and cool completely before decanting into storage containers. Refrigerated sauce keeps for several days. If freezing, use within 1 month.

MAKES 2 CUPS

Blurring the lines between sweet and savory, this modern bowl is a new favorite. With a satisfying base of coconut yogurt and cooked squash, it's a sophisticated addition to your next hors d'oeuvres plate. Serve with injera, raw vegetables, or eat straight out of your favorite bowl.

TROPIC OF THE HUDSON BOWL

½ seeded roast squash (kabocha, butternut or acorn)

½ cup coconut yogurt

1 tablespoon tahini

Himalayan pink salt, to taste

2 tablespoons hemp seeds

1 tablespoon pepitas

Freshly ground black pepper, to taste

Olive oil

Preheat the oven to 350°F. Brush the squash with olive oil, salt and pepper and lay cut side down on a baking sheet. Roast for 25 minutes and check to see if done. If not soft, roast for another 5 minutes and check again. Once cool enough to handle, remove flesh from skin and set aside to cool. Keep a little squash to the side to top your bowl with; the rest will go in the blender.

Add all but 2 tablespoons of the squash, the yogurt, tahini and salt to a high-speed blender and puree. Pour into your favorite bowl and top with the hemp seeds, pepitas, more salt (if needed), pepper, a tiny dash of oil and the reserved squash.

SERVES 2

Cindy's grandfather was an artist and potter who made most of his creations on an apple farm named White Cloud. Reminiscent of the pies and crumbles of our childhood, this modern take on a favorite dessert is nutrient-dense, low in sugar and delicious on the plate. Consider this dessert a love song to art, food and family.

WHITE CLOUD BAKE

1¼ cups gluten-free rolled oats

1 cup pumpkin seeds

¾ cup brown rice flour

1 tablespoon ground cardamom

1 teaspoon ground cinnamon

½ cup + ½ teaspoon coconut oil

2 teaspoons vanilla extract or 1 vanilla bean

½ cup + 1 tablespoon maple syrup

½ teaspoon Himalayan pink salt

½ teaspoon coconut oil

FILLING

2 cups roughly chopped apples and/or pears

½ cup dried golden berries

1½ teaspoons brown rice flour

1 tablespoon coconut sugar

½ teaspoon lemon zest

½ teaspoon cinnamon

¼ teaspoon ginger

STREUSEL TOPPING

¼ cup pumpkin seeds, roughly chopped

¼ cup gluten-free rolled oats

Preheat the oven to 350°F.

Combine the oats and pumpkin seeds in a food processor and blend until finely ground. Add the flour, cardamom, cinnamon and ½ cup of the oil, vanilla, syrup and salt and process until combined, scraping down the sides, if necessary. (If the dough seems too dry, add 1 tablespoon water.) Allow to rest for 30 minutes. Grease a 9 x 13-inch cake pan with the remaining ½ teaspoon of oil. Then, place three-quarters of the dough in the center of the pan. Firmly press the dough into the pan, covering the entire bottom surface of the pan evenly. Using a fork, make holes all over the dough. Bake for 10 minutes, then rotate and bake for an additional 5 minutes. Remove from the oven and lower the temperature to 325°F.

To make the filling: In a mixing bowl combine the apples and/or pears, berries, flour, sugar, lemon zest, cinnamon and ginger.

To make the streusel: In a small mixing bowl, place the remaining dough. Break it up into small pieces with your hands and then mix in the pumpkin seeds and oats.

To assemble: Transfer the filling directly on top of the baked crust in an even layer. Sprinkle the topping over the filling. Bake for 25 to 30 minutes, or until the filling begins to bubble and the streusel is golden brown.

SERVES 10 TO 15

This simple raw chocolate is made magical by the shen-supporting benefits of reishi. Use it as a canvas for adding High Vibrational toppings like bee pollen, goji berries or cacao nibs. Or keep it simple. Radiant beauty begins within.

HEAL ME CHOCOLATE

1 cup raw cacao powder

⅔ cup + 1 tablespoon coconut oil, melted, plus more if needed

½ cup unsweetened coconut flakes

⅓ cup maple syrup or coconut nectar

2 tablespoons reishi

½ teaspoon Himalayan pink salt

OPTIONAL TOPPINGS

Bee pollen

Cacao nibs

Goji berries

Fill a medium saucepan with water and bring to a boil over high heat.

Meanwhile, place all the ingredients into a food processor or high-speed blender and process until the coconut flakes have broken down and the mixture has become a thick paste. Transfer to a metal bowl and set on top of the boiling saucepan. Gently warm the chocolate, stirring often with a heatproof metal spatula, 1 to 2 minutes. The consistency should be a bit runny but thick enough to cover the back of a spoon. If the chocolate is too thick, add a bit more oil, 1 tablespoon at a time. Pour the chocolate in an even layer on a parchment-lined baking sheet. Sprinkle on the bee pollen (if using), cacao (if using) and berries (if using). Place the pan in the freezer to chill. Remove the pan after 30 minutes, and break the chocolate into chunks. Store in the refrigerator.

MAKES 4 CUPS

Cindy's husband, Laurent, knows his way around a crepe. The Paris native spent childhood summers in Brittany, where crepes are king. We love the earthy flavors of buckwheat and early autumn figs. Laurent loves the High Vibe nod to his motherland.

LOLO LOVES CREPES

2 cups buckwheat flour

½ cup cacao powder

1 teaspoon Himalayan pink salt

3½ cups filtered water

1 tablespoon ground flaxeeds

Coconut oil

COMPOTE

1 pound fresh figs, halved, or ½ pound dried

1 tablespoon fresh lemon juice

1 teaspoon lemon zest

2 tablespoons coconut sugar

2 tablespoons cacao powder

1 teaspoon vanilla extract (or ½ vanilla bean, scraped)

CHOCOLATE SAUCE

¼ cup coconut oil

¼ cup cacao powder

1 tablespoon lucuma powder

Cacao nibs

Sliced figs

Toasted hazelnuts

Om Chantilly (page 264)

In a large bowl, combine the flour, cacao, flaxseeds, salt and 3½ cups of the water. Allow to rest for 30 minutes or overnight.

To make the compote: Add the figs, lemon juice, lemon zest, sugar, cacao and vanilla to a medium saucepan. Place over medium heat and cook at a simmer, stirring often, for 30 minutes, or until the figs are broken down and most of the liquid has been absorbed. Remove from the heat and let cool.

To make the chocolate sauce: Warm the oil over a double boiler until liquefied. Whisk in the cacao and lucuma and stir well. Remove from the heat and set aside.

To make the crepes: Warm a bit of coconut oil in a nonstick skillet or crepe pan. Once melted, tilt the pan to cover the entire diameter of the skillet. Immediately pour in about ¼ cup of the batter. Very quickly, tilt the pan once more to cover the entire surface with batter. Return the skillet to the heat. Cook the crepe over medium-low heat until the edges begin to bubble and the bottom starts to release. Remove and continue with the rest of the batter.

To assemble: Place a crepe on a flat surface, drop ¼ cup of the compote in the center. Place on a serving plate. Drizzle chocolate sauce over the top, and serve with the cacao nibs, figs, hazelnuts and whipped cream.

MAKES 15 CREPES (USING AN 8-INCH PAN)

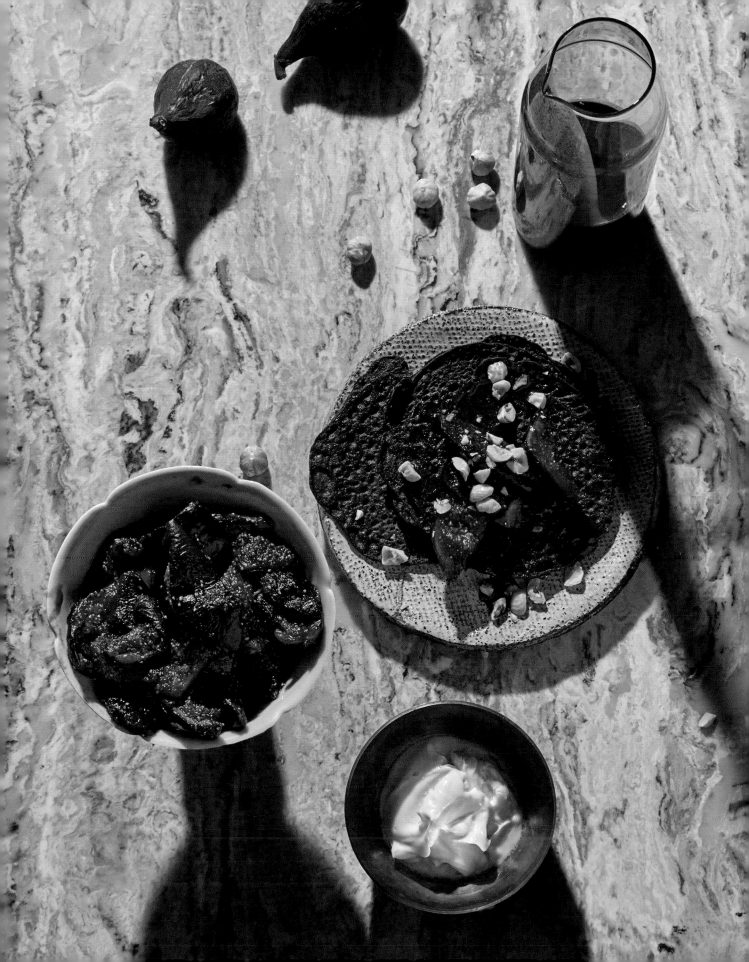

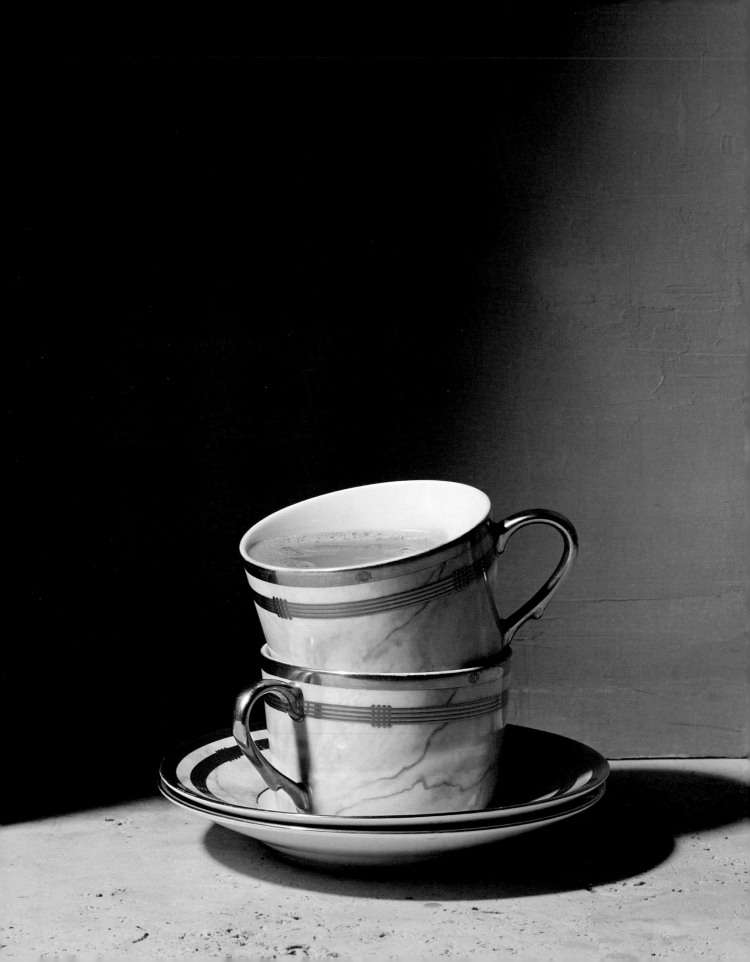

The official house drink of CAP Beauty draws its magic from the Taoist herb, he shou wu, used for centuries to deliver glowing skin, lustrous hair and long, strong nails. It's beyond delicious, and our customers can't get enough. Some even take one for the road.

THE BEAUTY ELIXIR

8 ounces nut or seed milk

½ teaspoon he shou wu

1 to 2 tablespoons tocotrienols

1 tablespoon coconut butter or The Daily Hit (page 217)

Heat the nut milk in a small saucepan until warm, but do not boil. Combine the milk with the he shou wu, tocotrienols and butter in a blender, and blend for a full minute. Pour into your favorite tea bowl or mug and drink it in.

SERVES 1

Roses are known to have the highest vibrational frequency of any flower, which could be one of the reasons why they're so universally loved. But, it also could be that they smell divine. Or, that they're delicious. This tea highlights their beauty, inside and out. Drink it in, and let beauty begin within.

HIGHEST VIBE ROSE TEA

Handful of fresh rose petals (see Note)

6 to 8 ounces filtered water

Green or herbal tea (optional)

Add a small handful of rose petals to your favorite green tea and brew as usual or steep straight up and sip all day long.

NOTE: It's vital to use carefully sourced roses as they are often sprayed and are not regulated as food. In New York City, try the Greenmarket. But make sure to check that they're not sprayed.

SERVES 1

THE RITUALS: LIGHT UP

THE WINTER SKIN PROGRAM

PERFORM: Twice daily, and as needed

WHAT YOU'LL NEED: Cleanser, toner and oil or moisturizer, plus an optional balm

DURATION: 5 to 10 minutes

Frigid temperatures and powerful heaters make for confused and challenged skin. Just like we dress for the cold by adding layers, we recommend this same tactic for skincare. Don't go out without your coat! Products that may feel heavy in the warmer months absorb quickly into parched skin and create a protective barrier from environmental stressors like the bitter wind and the freezing cold. The idea here is to keep your skin protected, nourished and hydrated. Depending on your level of dryness, this may mean applying *and reapplying* throughout the day. Adding nutrition at skin level is your baseline defense against damage.

Cleanse with an oil or cream cleanser, and massage it into your skin like you mean it. The more time you spend on this crucial step, the more benefits you'll see and feel. During the colder months, when we move less, boosting circulation is vital. Think of it as a mini trip to the spa, indulge yourself and get into it. Massage benefits you physically and mentally and creates truly radiant skin. We make a practice in all seasons to always cleanse at night and recommend assessing your skin in the morning to see if you truly need to cleanse. Sometimes just a quick rinse with warm and cool water will do the trick.

While your skin is still damp, mist generously with toner. As we've said in earlier chapters, today's hydrosols are nothing like the astringent and stripping toners from 30 years ago. A good toner should hydrate, nourish and even, in some cases, exfoliate. And, they'll allow your oils, balms and serums to penetrate more deeply. This is vital during these very dry months.

Alternatively, you can add your toner to an oil or moisturizer. Mix together in your hand and apply to your face while still damp. By emulsifying the two, you create a bespoke product that will sink more readily into the skin. Again, winter calls for deep hydration, and this is one of the best ways to get it.

Layer on as many sources of nutrients and hydration as you want or need. Including a balm is an option for very dry or mature skin. We also like to keep bottles of hydrosols close at hand, on the nightstand, in our bags and at our desks. Mist anytime inspiration strikes. It's great over makeup, too. We mist ourselves all day. Even during meetings. Let's just call it research.

Layer up. Your winter skin will thank you.

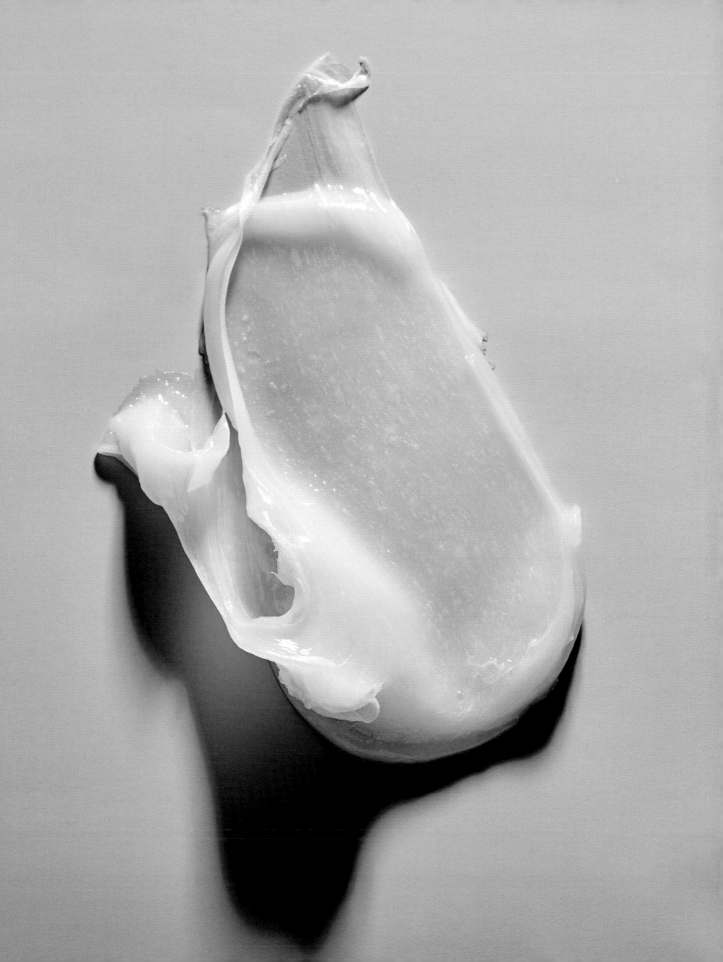

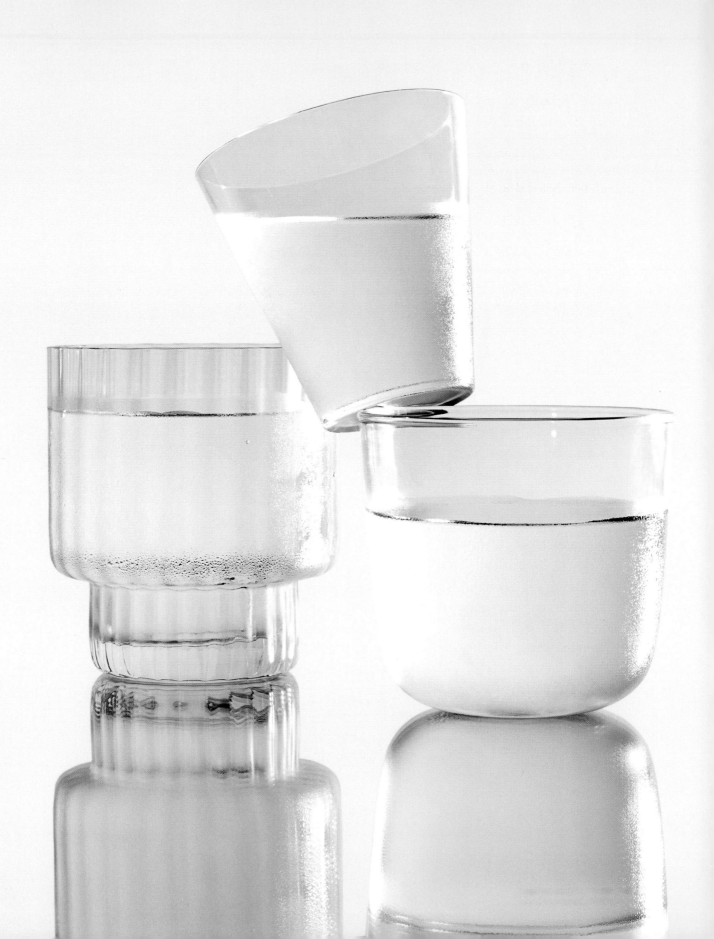

HYDRATE TO HEAL

Drink it in. We're all too familiar with the ubiquitous eight glasses a day. Water is life, and we all benefit from drinking enough. We know you've heard it before, but before you turn the page, hear us out. Hydration is key, and every aspect of your health will benefit. Including your skin. So many of our customers come to us in winter months complaining of dry and dehydrated skin. Here's what to do.

Find a glass you truly love, and consider it your portal to hydration. Keep it handy at home and at work. Add lemon, if that helps. Another great tip is to start the day with a *big* glass of filtered water with lemon. This alkalizes your system and jump starts your digestion, setting you up for a day of healthy habits. It's especially important to do this if you are inclined to reach for a cup of coffee before eating.

Water should be filtered or from the spring, but we urge you to rethink the plastic bottle. There are great options for filters, from an under-sink installed unit to a ceramic countertop vessel or high-style pitcher to a chic water bottle that travels with you.

Drink all day, but not with or right before a meal, as that can make for more complicated digestion. And, wait about an hour after eating to hit the bottle again.

While lemons are a common addition, we also like to spike our water (especially a well-sourced sparkling mineral water) with sea buckthorn pureed berries. It's *super* tart and bright orange, and makes a great alternative to an evening cocktail. Sea buckthorn berries are one of nature's highest sources of omega-7 fatty acids, also known as the beauty nutrient. Sea buckthorn berry oil is even used topically to treat burn victims, because it's a potent anti-inflammatory. Taking it internally encourages healing and hydration from within. So, raise a glass.

WINTER PRODUCT RECOMMENDATIONS

CLEANSER: Pai Camellia and Rose Gentle Hydrating Cleanser, de Mamiel Restorative Cleansing Balm, S. W. Basics Cleanser

HYDROSOL: Tata Harper Hydrating Floral Essence, Leahlani Bohemian Ruby Balancing Toner, Elaa Moonlight Mist Celestial Facial Toner

MOISTURIZER: Odacité Beautiful Day Moisturizer, Honey Girl Face and Eye Crème, Dr. Alkaitis Day Crème

SERUM: Vintner's Daughter Active Botanical Serum, de Mamiel Winter Facial Oil, In Fiore Complexe de Fleur

OTHER GOOD STUFF: One Love Organics Skin Savior, May Lindstrom The Honey Mud, Henné Luxury Lip Balm, Julisis Eyemulsion

NUTRIENT MASKS

PERFORM: Once
or twice a week

WHAT YOU'LL NEED:
A ready-made mask
or a bowl, a brush,
manuka honey, tea
and other ingredients
of your choosing

DURATION:
10 minutes
to an hour

Another way to add hydration and nutrition to challenged winter skin is to incorporate masks into your routine. We love the ritual of masking, as it embodies true self care and forces us to take a break from constantly "doing." Beauty begins when we flood our bodies, both inside and out, with nutrient dense ingredients from plants, minerals and the hive. As we've stated before, there are masks for every skin concern, masks that draw out impurities, masks that soothe and masks that deliver high levels of nutrition. The winter months call for exfoliation, hydration and healing. There are plenty of premade masks to address these needs, but you can also blend your own. A great base is the all-powerful and healing manuka honey. Moisturizing, cleansing, exfoliating and a natural anti-bacterial, this star ingredient is a beauty hero. Add to that any number of ingredients tailored to your needs, and you can't go wrong, so alchemize away. Here's our mini guide to making masks:

Add 2 tablespoons manuka honey to a small mixing bowl. If manuka honey isn't available to you, find the best quality raw and local honey you can find. The farmer's market is sometimes a great source. Brew some green tea or matcha or, for very sensitive skin, try chamomile. Slowly add about 1 teaspoon of the tea and stir to combine. Be careful not to overthin the mask. Then, pick and choose from the ingredients below to create your custom mask. Blend together, brush onto your freshly cleaned skin and take a rest. This is also a great time to take a bath. The humidity will further activate the honey. Leave on your face for 10 minutes or longer (you can leave it on up to 45 minutes if you wish). Then, rinse with warm to cool water, and gently pat your skin dry with a clean towel. Follow with an oil or moisturizer of your choice, but keep it simple. This is not the time for your most active and intense products. Your skin is fresh and clean. Let it be, and enjoy its luster.

Here are the mix-ins for winter masks:

TOCOTRIENOLS. This rice-bran soluble powder is light and airy, and it's packed with bioavailable vitamins D and E. If you live in a northern climate, your skin is most likely lacking vitamin D. Feed yourself. Mix 1 tablespoon into your base for a nutrient rich mask.

ALGAE. Chlorella, spirulina and E3Live are three nutritional powerhouses that deliver chlorophyll and oxygenate the skin. Look for single ingredient powders or a blend. E3Live also comes as a frozen liquid. If you're using this form, thaw slightly and pour a teaspoon or so off the top and blend with your mask. Otherwise, simply add a teaspoon or so of powder. Your mask will turn a satisfying shade of deep green and will mineralize and alkalize your skin.

100 PERCENT SHEA BUTTER. Richly hydrating and emollient, this old school and high hippie ingredient takes on even the most severely dry skin. When you're really parched, this is the ingredient to add. Straight from the jar, shea butter is almost solid and difficult to incorporate. Start with ½ teaspoon, and, using clean hands, warm until soft. Add this into your bowl and continue to blend. Then, reap the riches.

MATCHA. Any chance we have to use matcha, we use it. Even on the skin. Loaded with antioxidants and vitamin C, this Japanese delicacy translates perfectly to the face by encouraging a reduction in inflammation and evening out skin tone. Teatime for your skin.

THE WINTER BATH

'Tis the season for diving deep and staying put. Our favorite indulgence for honoring this time of committed self care is a warm winter bath. Let this ritual rule your week. Kerrilynn likes to schedule a regular bath night each week, but don't shy away from spontaneity, from more frequent baths to soaking it in on the daily. You can make this as simple or as ceremonial as you like.

For a hydrating and nourishing soak, use your favorite body oil or simply use coconut or jojoba oil. While you run the warm bath, stand outside of the tub and give yourself a full body massage, generously working the oil into your skin. This is particularly nice if you warm the oil beforehand. To do this, decant enough oil into a glass kitchen jar and submerge the jar in a pot of hot water. Be careful when removing as it will be hot and possibly slippery. If you use enough oil for your massage, there's no need to add additional oil to the bath. Get in the tub (carefully!) and relax. Use this time to meditate, listen to your favorite podcast or just be. This is your time. Lock the door.

When you're finished, drain the tub and be sure to thoroughly wipe it down, as the oil will make it very slippery. You won't need to moisturize. Have a clean towel or bedsheet on hand, and wrap yourself up for the night. Sweet dreams.

PERFORM:
Once or twice a week or every night

WHAT YOU'LL NEED:
Body oil, a kitchen jar and a clean towel

DURATION:
20 minutes to an hour

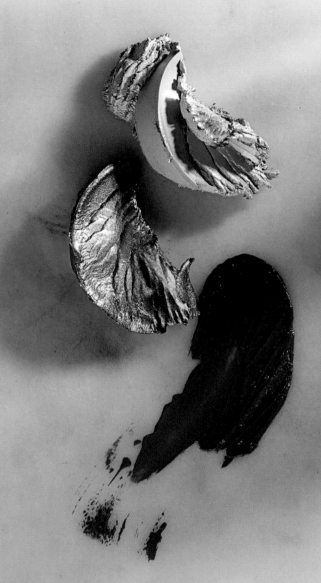

THE MAKEUP PALETTE

The metallic and magical glow of the holidays inspires our makeup choices for the season. Paired with the classic red lip, we are one part alight and one part afoot. Tawny golds and shimmery taupes are grounded by a hit of hardworking red. Embrace the extremes of the season. Let the color you add light your way.

SALUTE THE SUN

During the dark days of winter when sunlight is scarce, we welcome it in with salutation. The classic yogic series, The Sun Salutation, raises heat in the body and calls to mind the power of our mighty sun. Start each morning with this practice to raise your vibration and welcome the day.

Seasoned yogis, you know the drill. For all others, here's how to do it: If you're feeling rusty, start by gently stretching out your body. Some easy forward bends are great. As you bend over, grab opposite elbows and let your head and arms succumb to gravity. Feel free to rock a bit and let your body lead the way. When you're ready to begin, stand at the front of your mat, hands in prayer at your chest. Inhale deeply, and lift your arms to a high prayer above the head, looking upward as you do. Swan dive forward to a deep forward bend and, if you can, reach your fingertips to the floor in front of you. From there straighten your spine and lift the head, chin and chest parallel with the floor. This is called preparing the spine. Release and step back to Plank pose. Plank pose resembles the top of a pushup. For an added challenge you can hold Plank pose for a few breaths, engaging the core as you do. Then, slowly bend the elbows without sinking the hips or collapsing your core for a yogi pushup. The elbows should stay at 90 degrees so your body does not drop all the way to the floor. Now pull yourself forward into Upward Dog, extend your arms, arch your back and roll over your toes so that you're resting on the tops of your feet. Your head will be lifted. When you've reached the full extent of this position, lead with your hips and find Downward Facing Dog, stretching your heels toward the floor. Stay here for five deep breaths, and then step or jump forward between your hands and return to the starting position. Repeat this series three or four more times or build from there. Sacred practices encourage 108 repetitions. Obviously, this isn't for every day. But, a few rounds of this practice in the morning will work out the kinks and warm you up for the day ahead.

PERFORM: Daily

WHAT YOU'LL NEED: Comfortable clothes and a yoga mat or clear space on the floor

DURATION: 5 to 15 minutes

BREATH OF FIRE

PERFORM: Daily

WHAT YOU'LL NEED:
Comfortable
clothes and a seat
on the floor

DURATION:
1 to 3 minutes

Get stoked. This basic pranayama practice is powerful for heating your body, moving energy, and cleansing your respiratory channels. Just 1 minute creates a profound shift. Practice anytime to revive and recharge yourself.

Sit on the floor in Virasana pose, or a cross-legged position. Begin by inhaling deeply and exhaling completely. Repeat two more times, and then take a comfortable breath in to about three-quarters of your capacity. Rest your hands on your knees, with your palms up and your thumbs and index fingers touching. Or, for a more challenging pose, raise your arms in a V above your head with your palms facing up. Begin sharp, fast, forceful and conscious exhales. Do not focus on the inhale. This will happen naturally. With each rapid exhale, pull your abdomen in and up. Repeat for 100 breaths or set a timer and go for a minute. When complete, take a deep inhalation, hold the breath, and apply chin and root lock. (Chin lock, also known as Jalandhara, is the simple act of closing the throat by tilting the chin toward the chest. Root lock or Mula Bandha is the practice of lifting and tightening the perineum and sex organs.) Exhale and repeat. Take note of how you feel before and after this practice. Its effects can be profound. Notice the shift, and enjoy the lightness of being.

SEEING (INFRA)RED

When nature's forces work against us, our mission for the season is to turn up the heat. Stepping inside a warm sauna has obvious appeal during the coldest months, but its benefits are far more profound than just the temporary warmth. Any sauna will assist in detoxification, by encouraging sweating, but far infrared saunas take their mission higher. They feel noticeably less hot than a classic sauna, but heat us from within, creating benefits on a cellular level. Far infrared light warms us in a manner similar to the sun. A session in a far infrared sauna increases serotonin, reduces cortisol, burns calories, stimulates collagen production, increases flexibility, oxygenates the cells and improves circulation. Some have even used far infrared saunas to clear up breakouts and boost skin health. And, if all that isn't enough, infrared light creates a more efficient release of toxins. Seek one out to sweat it out.

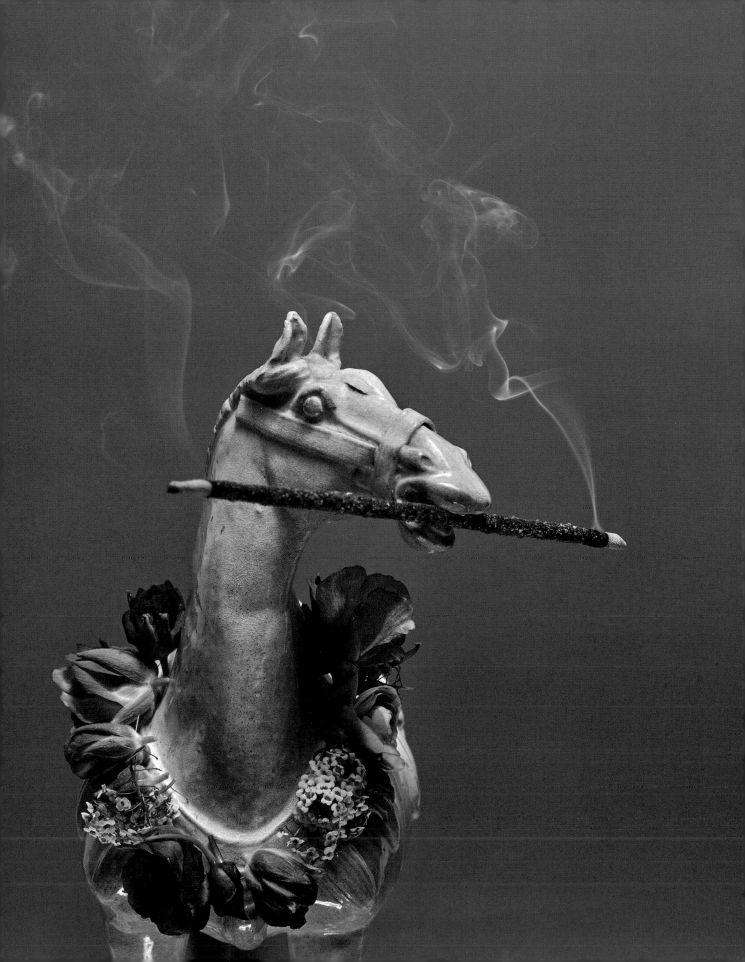

IMMUNITY COMMUNITY

Don't go it alone. There's much talk these days of the complex and curious microbiome and the legions of bacteria that inhabit our bodies. We're learning more each day about the role of these bacteria, and their sway on everything from digestion to immunity. They even affect our brains, controlling cravings and our ability to focus. The key here is to make sure that we create the right environment for the good bacteria (or probiotics) to thrive, while discouraging the proliferation of the less friendly type. Here are some basic tips and tricks for building up your biome.

CHOOSE FERMENTS. Adding fermented foods to your daily intake will increase the presence of good bacteria and promote a healthy immune system. Foods that are naturally fermented like raw sauerkraut, kombucha and miso include a wide spectrum of naturally occurring good bacteria. Remember that "Diversity on the plate equals diversity in the gut," so mix it up and get creative. You can find an incredible selection of fermented vegetables at your local health food store, or make your own. We love the book *Wild Fermentation* by Sandor Katz as a place to begin.

PREACTIVATE. Another strategy to employ to encourage a healthy microbiome is to choose foods that feed the good bacteria. These are known as prebiotics and are a type of fiber found in certain roots and other fruits and vegetables. Raw garlic, raw dandelions, chicory root and Jerusalem artichokes, cooked or raw, are some of the highest sources. We like to roast a batch of Jerusalem artichokes to have on hand for the week. Toss into salads or have as a snack. (But be careful—Jerusalem artichokes can cause intestinal gas, so start slow!)

TAKE A PILL. Adding a good quality probiotic to your supplement program is a great idea as well. We always favor whole food sources of our vital nutrients but believe in adding this in as insurance. Some can survive without refrigeration, so look for those if you're traveling. And, choose a probiotic with multiple strains. Remember, diversity rules.

KEEP IT DIRTY TO KEEP IT CLEAN. Avoid antibacterial soaps, detergents and gels. These can destroy your precious bacteria and compromise your health. And, while it may not be possible in the winter months, literally getting dirty and walking barefoot will also introduce these friendly bacteria to your system.

SOS. We understand that there may be critical times when an antibiotic is needed. Because these drugs do not differentiate between good and bad bacteria, they can ironically wipe you clean of your best defenses. When you've completed your course of treatment, give your gut some extra love. Rebuild your front lines with the foods and practices above.

SHED THE LAYERS

The pen is mightier than the sword. And, this doesn't just apply to diplomacy. Write it out to get it out and liberate your mind. The simple act of putting pen to paper has profound benefits. We like the raw, unedited, stream-of-consciousness, for-your-eyes-only variety. This practice can relieve you of obsessive thinking and gets your thoughts on the page and out of your head. Do it daily. You'll get to know yourself, recognize patterns and purge your mind of clutter. A clean slate awaits.

PERFORM: Daily

WHAT YOU'LL NEED:
A journal and a pen

DURATION:
5 to 10 minutes

RESOLUTION REVOLUTION

Flip the script. Ditch the list you write every year. Simplify and distill these never-ending goals into one word you want to embody. Let it be your North Star. We realize that this shirks the conventional advice to get specific with your resolutions. But, we've found these overarching themes to be vastly more powerful and catalyzing. When life becomes busy, and your mind becomes cluttered, having one word to reference brings clarity and peace. Decisions become easier and more in line with your values. And, remember, it's the little things we do each day that create true change.

Pick a word that resonates with you, and watch how elegantly it applies to every area of your life. When we first started this practice, this surprised us. A seemingly vague concept like "spacious" became a physical, mental, emotional and spiritual touchstone. From Pigeon pose to a complex spreadsheet to a charged conversation with a lover, this word offers guidance and direction. Don't overthink this. The word you're drawn to is your word. Make it yours.

CRYSTALS FOR MOVING FORWARD

These are the stones we keep on hand to propel ourselves forward, to activate change, and get things done.

SMOKY QUARTZ: This moody stone clears the way for positive thoughts, propelling you toward your goals.

LABRADORITE: This mystical beauty cleanses your aura to prime you for making magic.

PYRITE: This architectural gem encourages the completion of projects and acts as a cheerleader seeing you through to the finish.

CITRINE: Ethereal and bright, citrine brings joy and magnifies your energy and power.

BLACK TOURMALINE: Stress takes a hit from this black beauty. Block negative energy and support your adrenals.

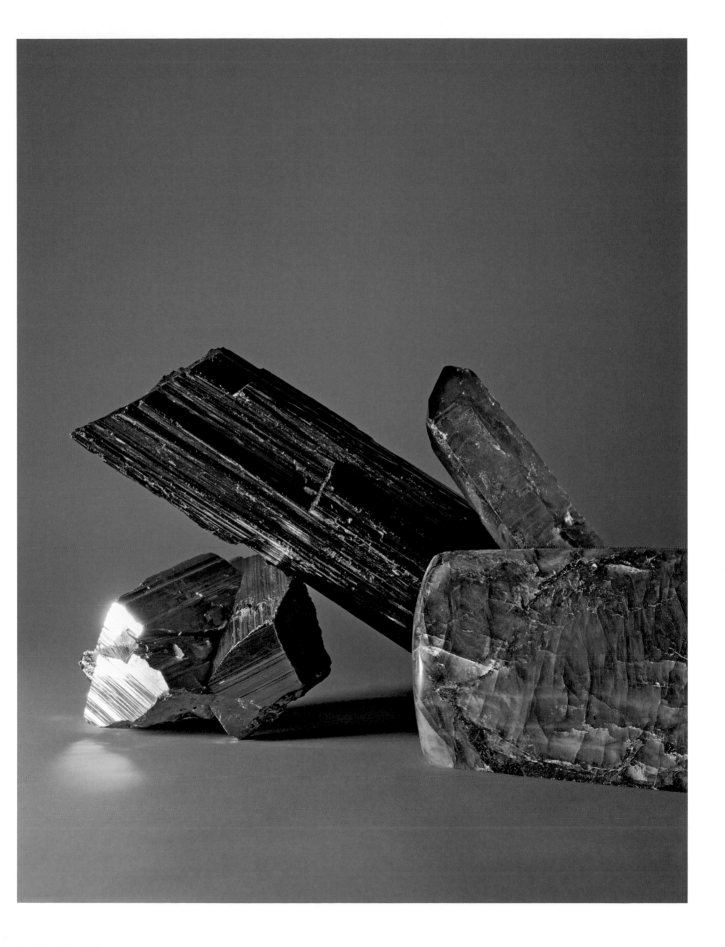

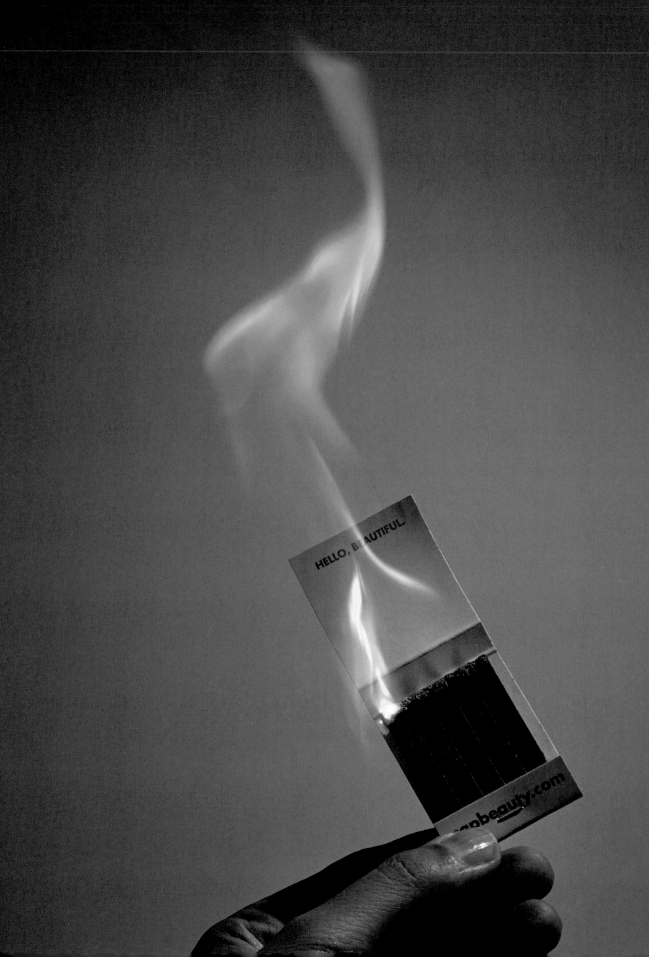

FIRE BUILDING

Home is where the hearth is. We talk a lot about building fire from within. And, we also love the fireplace variety. If you're lucky enough to have access to a fireplace, by all means, use it. Sometimes, this task may seem daunting, like more than you care to take on, but this ritualistic and primal act grounds us and connects us to the elements. The scent, the sounds and its emanating warmth change our surroundings like nothing else we know.

To build a raging one, we go for the upside-down method. Start with the largest logs at the bottom, with no space in between. Next add slightly smaller logs, again with no space in between. Keep piling on smaller and smaller wood in the same fashion, and then top with crumpled paper and kindling. Light the fire from the top, and bask in its glorious warmth.

Let this be your winter backdrop for meditating, writing, dining, loving and drinking tea.

WORD UP

What you see is what you get. One of our favorite practices to stay motivated and inspired is to seek and surround ourselves with intelligent and moving quotes. You can literally search "inspiring quotes," and however *Saturday Night Live* "Deep Thoughts" this might feel, you're sure to find some brilliance that resonates with you.

Now, you have a design project. Type or write these words and place them where you'll see them the most. On the fridge, the bathroom mirror, on a card in your wallet or by your desk. Read them, absorb them and let them work their magic. Consistency pays off.

THE HOLIDAY JOURNAL

Take the daze out of holidays. We love this time of year, but it's no secret that this season can put a lot on our plates. Gift giving, entertaining and traveling can challenge even the most organized. Rein it all in with a holiday journal. Keep track of everything from holiday tipping to budgets to parties to menus and seasonal recipes. The idea here is to have it all concisely in one place, allowing you to reference previous years and create ease around the season. A little planning goes a long way and keeps stress at bay.

We like to sit down shortly after Thanksgiving with a tonic drink or tea and start planning. Who will you buy for this year? How much will you spend? When will cross-country packages need to ship? Anything you can do to systematize it will bring joy back into the season.

PERFORM:
As needed

WHAT YOU'LL NEED:
A binder, pen, printed templates and envelopes for receipts

DURATION:
As needed

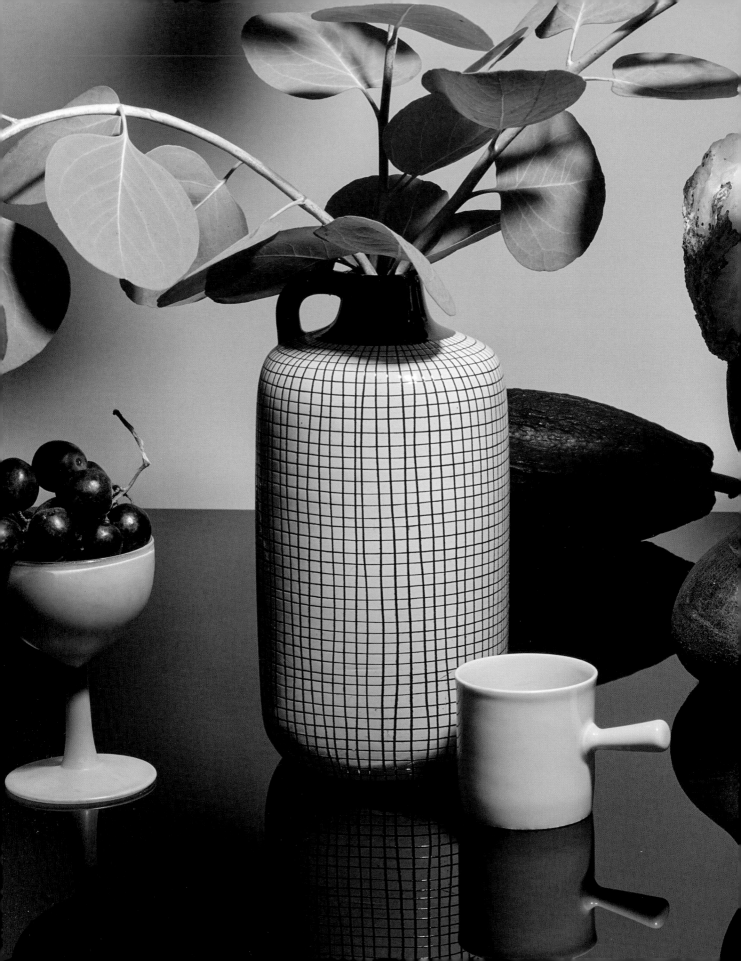

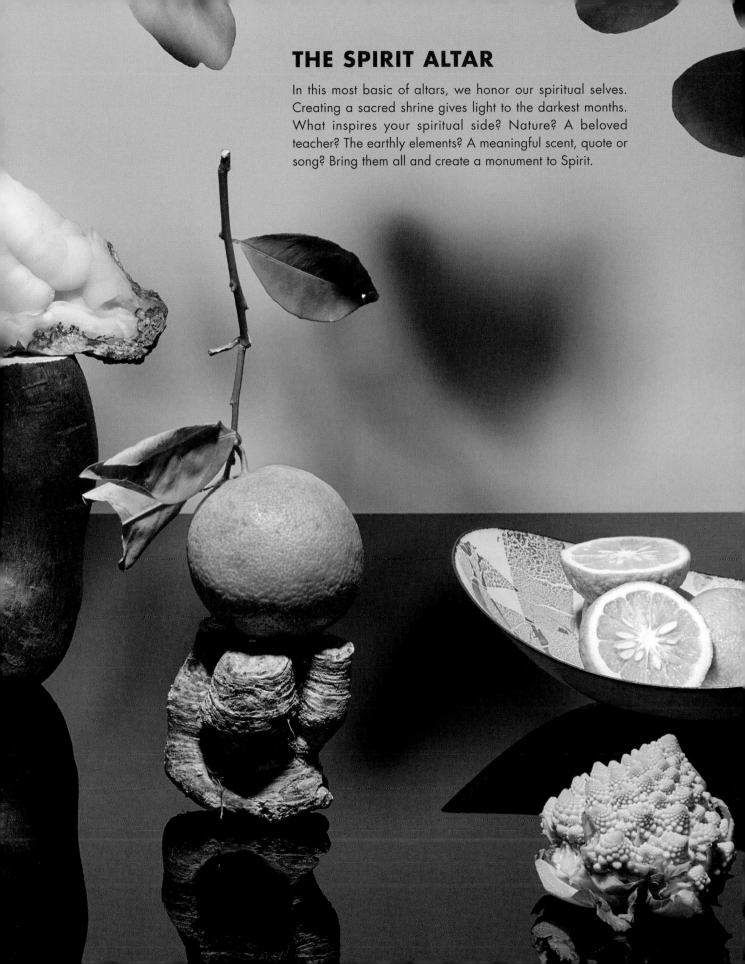

THE SPIRIT ALTAR

In this most basic of altars, we honor our spiritual selves. Creating a sacred shrine gives light to the darkest months. What inspires your spiritual side? Nature? A beloved teacher? The earthly elements? A meaningful scent, quote or song? Bring them all and create a monument to Spirit.

THE WINTER BEDROOM

Create a sanctuary for rest, ritual and love. We look to Northern Europe and our Scandinavian friends for inspiration and a modern approach to winter nesting. *Hygge*, the Scandinavian pursuit of coziness during the dark winter months, is an art and makes the most of short days and minimal light. We use this as our North Star, and build a winter bedroom that invites the deepest sleep and the strongest connection to ourselves and our lovers. Think layers: textiles, books, incense, natural light, crystals and botanicals. Get warm with a perfectly brewed tea or tonic in a favorite handmade mug. Indulge in a great pair of Japanese socks. Cover your bed with organic heavyweight linen, or add layers of beauty and warmth with your favorite blankets. We love a considered maximalist approach, adding texture but only allowing in objects that you truly love. Let each piece enrich your experience. Edit out the rest. Stay home, and stay close.

COOK AND CONNECT

Nothing brings people together like a great meal. We love the ritual of a standing date, one that all your friends know. Make it at regular intervals, like the first Sunday of every month, and let the tradition grow. When friends know that there's an open door and a great meal awaiting, they'll make their way over to share the day. Keep it open house–style with loose hours. Welcome kids and pets and out-of-town guests. The more, the merrier.

We look to the Brits and their traditional Sunday roasts, but our ovens are packed with plants and life-giving nourishment. Plan to serve foods that don't require last-minute prep. A pot of chili, a casserole, room-temperature salads and High Vibrational snacks. Cindy is a big believer in having a few stand-by recipes that she serves at almost every gathering. Her friends have grown to look forward to these tried-and-true treats, and it saves her time and stress. This Sunday gathering is about ease, grace and connecting to friends, not about testing complicated recipes. Keep it simple but inspired, and enjoy the company. You may even inspire a friend or two to start their own traditions.

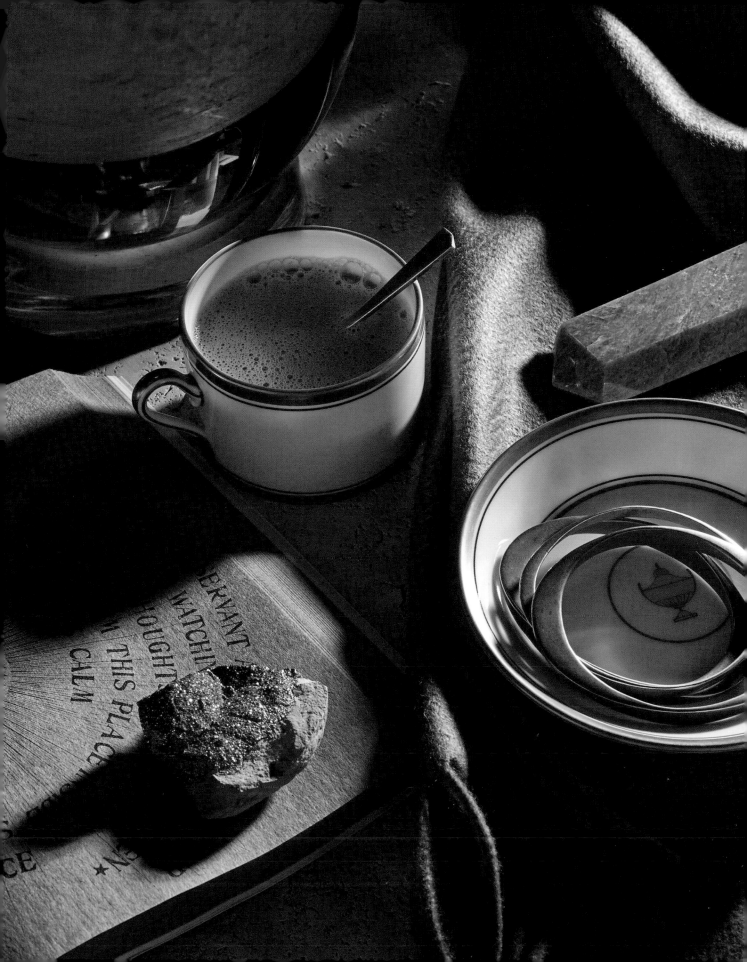

GIVING BACK

Give it to get it. Set the tone for the new year by creating a habit of giving. We know that after an indulgent December, many of us feel limited financially. But think beyond the checkbook. We all have time (whether we think so or not), and we all have causes that resonate. If you know someone doing great and important work, share the love by promoting their cause on social media and otherwise spread the word. If you have a friend who's having a difficult time, invite her to dinner. Walk dogs, or visit a nursing home. Help someone find a job. Use your network for good. Of course, writing a check or spending the day at a soup kitchen always works. But, get creative about how you can help. It might just surprise you how a simple act can profoundly help someone. The times when your resources are the most limited are the times to dig the deepest. You'll find your power there and create a vibration that will reverberate beyond yourself. Let it be a habit.

A DAY IN THE LIFE:
A WINTER'S TALE

RISE UP, PART THE BLINDS, AND LET WINTER'S QUIET LIGHT WAKE you. Be still. Scan your mind for what you feel most grateful for, and hold these things dear. Now, ask the Universe for what you need. Ask out loud, and be courageous. Trust that these things are coming your way. They are. Bring your body and mind to a place of meditation, whatever your practice. Set a timer. Or not. Focus on your breath, your mantra, or let yourself be guided. Wake gently from your meditative state. Welcome the world (and your lover or kids) slowly. Stretch it out, then head to the kitchen. Down a glass of filtered water with your probiotics. Drink it in. Your body's thirsty. Heat a pot of water for a warming alkalizing tonic. It can be as simple as lemon water. Or, prepare your favorite morning brew. Whatever gets you going. Add coconut oil to slow the release of caffeine into your gentle system. If you're having coffee, be sure to drink a big glass of lemon water first. Use your favorite mug. Surround yourself with beauty. Put on a favorite playlist, find your favorite chair and savor the morning. Then, get your body moving. A run, spin or fast session of HIIT is all you need to get your blood flowing and your mind sharp. Off to wash up. But, before you step into the shower, give yourself a good rub with a rich and decadent body oil. A few extra minutes of massage won't hurt. Step in and rinse away your hard-earned sweat and any excess oil. The steam from the shower and your massage will reveal your softest and most nourished skin. You can spend a few extra minutes conditioning your hair as well. When you step out of the shower, you may not need any additional moisturizer. But if you do, layer it on.

Wrap yourself in a clean and cozy towel or your favorite robe. Stay warm. Head back to the kitchen for a warming bowl of Amaranth Congee (page 216), or treat yourself to Himalayan High Cacao Oats (page 221), another tonic for the road perhaps and any supplements you take with food. Off to work or wherever your day takes you. The train is a great time to read, or listen to a favorite podcast. Take advantage of this downtime, then get present with whatever you're doing. Let lunchtime be me time. Put down the phone. Take the extra steps to ensure that you get a healthy meal. If your energy is lagging in the afternoon, try a matcha. Drink it in, and let the calm focus wash over you. Wrap up your day and greet the evening. The magic hour awaits. Light a candle, turn on the tunes and set the stage for a perfect night in. A warming meal. A book or movie or bath. Time with your lover (maybe that's you). Meditate once more, and get to bed early. There's lots to get to tomorrow.

STOKE YOUR FIRE

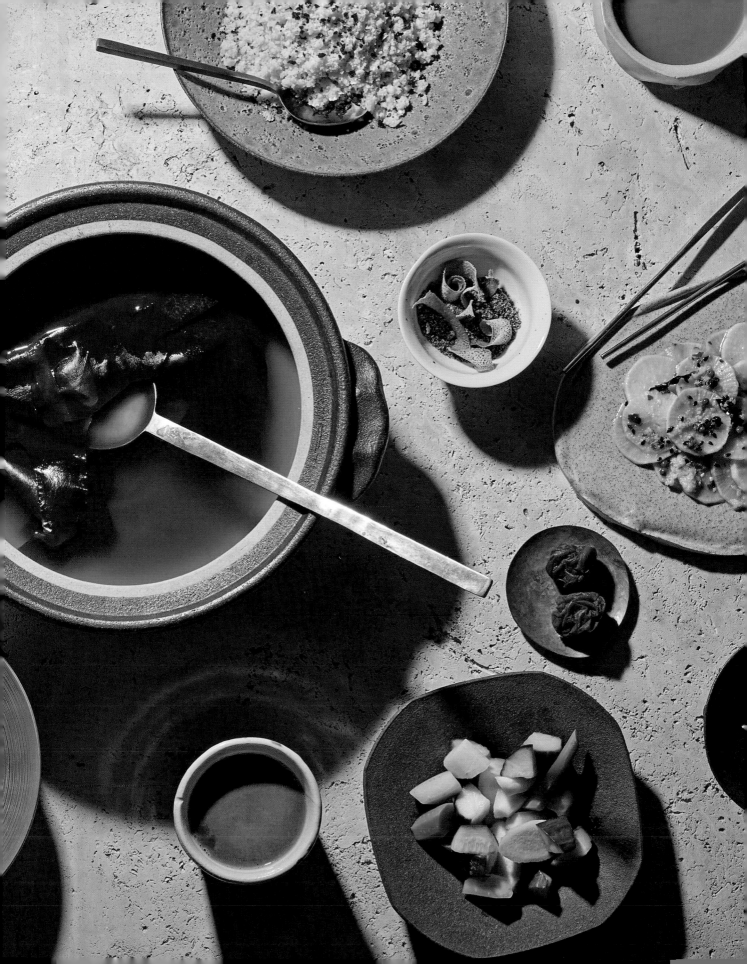

SHARE THE LOVE:
GOOD MORNING, TOKYO

An elegant and uncommon start to the day, Japanese breakfast is one of our favorites. Invite your Japanese food-loving friends for a salty-and-savory morning meal. Once again, we rely on the power of plants to deliver the deep-sea umami flavor that we crave.

HERE'S HOW TO DO IT: Like with so many of our parties, this breakfast asks guests to build their own bowls. Offer a basic morning miso alongside the toppings and treasures you love. Pull out your best wabi-sabi ceramics, your wooden boards and your favorite chopsticks and spoons. Good morning, Tokyo.

We like this party for a smaller group. Four to six people works best.

Miso Happy
(page 218)

SIDES
Cauliflower Rice
(below)

Brown rice, cooked

Asian Gravlax
(opposite)

Avocados

Nori sheets

Holy Herbs Schichimi
(page 266)

Umeboshi plums, sliced

Tamari

Radishes, finely sliced

Stewed nori

Pickled Vegetables
(opposite)

Sesame seeds, toasted

Taste of Tomoko
(page 266)

Dulse flakes

CAULIFLOWER COCONUT RICE

1 head cauliflower

1 tablespoon coconut oil

2 tablespoons tamari or coconut aminos (optional)

½ tablespoon sesame oil (optional)

Holy Herbs Schichimi (page 266; optional)

Taste of Tomoko (page 266; optional)

Grate the cauliflower on a box grater or add to a food processor and process until the cauliflower resembles rice. Heat the coconut oil in a large pot over medium heat and add the cauliflower. Cover and let steam, stirring occasionally, for 5 to 6 minutes, or until soft. Remove from the heat and add the tamari or aminos (if using), sesame oil (if using), Holy Herbs Schichimi and Taste of Tomoko.

SERVES 4 AS A SIDE DISH

ASIAN GRAVLAX

1 medium daikon radish, peeled

½ cup olive oil

½ cup grapeseed oil

1 teaspoon sesame oil

1 teaspoon salt

1 teaspoon coconut sugar

½ teaspoon brown rice vinegar

1 teaspoon tamari

½ teaspoon whole sansho peppercorns

½ teaspoon whole white peppercorns

½ teaspoon Holy Herbs Schichimi (page 266)

½ teaspoon whole black peppercorns

1 teaspoon black sesame seeds

1 teaspoon white sesame seeds

1 tablespoon grated ginger

2 tablespoons dulse

4 strips lemon zest

Preheat the oven to 300°F.

Slice the radishes into ¼-inch slices on a mandoline. Place the radish slices in a single even layer in a deep baking dish. Cover with olive, grapeseed and sesame oil, making sure there is enough to completely submerge the turnips. If not, add a bit more oil, if needed, up to ½ cup. Add the remaining ingredients and press down into the oil. Cook for 1 hour. Allow to cool, then refrigerate for 3 hours or overnight. Remove the slices from brine, making sure to brush off any spices.

MAKES 1 CUP OR SERVES 2

PICKLED VEGETABLES

5 carrots, cut into ½-inch pieces

1 large daikon radish, cut into ½-inch pieces

1 large cucumber, cut into ½-inch pieces

2 cups apple cider vinegar

1 chile

1 (1-inch) piece of ginger

Tamari or coconut aminos

6 peppercorns

Add the carrots, radish and cucumber into a 1-quart sterilized, glass jar. In a large saucepan over medium-high heat, bring the vinegar, chile, ginger, tamari or aminos and peppercorns to a boil, then remove from the heat and allow to cool. Pour the liquid brine on top of the vegetables and seal tightly. These will last for a week in your fridge.

MAKES 4 CUPS OR 1 QUART

Our brilliant and incomparable food stylist, Victoria Granof, introduced us to the power of congee over breakfast once, and we were hooked. The perfect canvas for toppings on repeat, this savory or sweet bowl is ripe for creation. Make it yours.

AMARANTH CONGEE

4 or 5 strips wakame

½ cup amaranth, rinsed

2 cups water or Kombu *Dashi* (page 264)

1 teaspoon grated fresh ginger

¼ teaspoon Himalayan pink salt

1½ teaspoons tamari

TOPPINGS (OPTIONAL)

Toasted sesame oil

Toasted sesame seeds

Scallions

Fermented vegetables and chiles

Julienned radishes

Lacto-Fermented Hot Sauce (page 256)

In a small bowl, soak the wakame in water for 10 minutes, or until rehydrated. Set aside.

Add the amaranth, water or dashi, ginger and salt in a large saucepan over medium high heat and bring to a boil. Reduce the heat to low, and simmer until most of the water has been absorbed and the amaranth is cooked through. Remove from heat and stir in the tamari. Drain the wakame and fold it in. Transfer to a large serving bowl and add toppings, as desired.

SERVES 2

A warming and grounding start to the day. Easy on digestion, this break-fast bowl sets you up for whatever the day may bring, and the thermo-genic spices have been known to boost metabolism. We like to add lots of citrus juice to make it bright. Serve the dhal on its own or over greens. You can also thin with water to make a soup. It's also great for lunch or dinner. It gets better over time, so make enough for leftovers. Fuel your fire.

GROUND DOWN DHAL

2 tablespoons coconut oil or The Daily Hit (below)

1 yellow onion, sliced

1 (2-inch) piece of ginger, peeled and minced

2 cloves garlic, smashed

1 tablespoon turmeric, fresh or dried

1 dried chile de arbol or other dried chile

1 teaspoon freshly ground black pepper

1 teaspoon salt

1 teaspoon coriander seeds

1 cup red lentils

4 cups filtered water

½ cup coconut milk (optional)

Lemon or lime juice, to taste

Warm the oil over medium heat in large, heavy bottomed pot. Add the onion, ginger, garlic, turmeric, chile, black pepper, salt and coriander seeds, and sauté until the onions are translucent and the mixture forms a pastelike consistency. Add the lentils, and stir to combine. Add the water and coconut milk (if using). Turn up the heat, bring to a boil and then turn down the heat and let simmer for 15 to 20 minutes, or until cooked through. Stir frequently, as split lentils cook quickly and have a tendency to stick to the bottom of the pan. The lentils will start to break down and the mixture will thicken. Remove from the heat and generously add lemon or lime juice.

SERVES 4

THE DAILY HIT

CBD is gaining momentum as an ingredient to take note of. Believed to decrease inflammation, encourage calm in the body and mind and take the edge off the stress of daily life, this is one of our new favorite foods to incorporate daily. Our natural, non-psychoactive blend takes it higher and incorporates adaptogenic herbs for focus, good mood and immune sup-port. A hit on your salad, in your smoothie or even laced in your coffee will get you soaring. Fly high, free bird.

It's always Japan for us, especially when it comes to food. Try Miso Happy for breakfast, and get in tune with one of the most elevated (and healthy) cultures around. We rely on its warming ingredients and ritualistic preparation to tune us in on a cold winter morning. Welcome your day with grace. *Arigato.*

MISO HAPPY

4 cups filtered water

1 (6-inch) piece of kombu

4 tablespoons miso

½ cup rehydrated wakame

2 tablespoons tamari, plus more if needed

1 carrot, finely sliced

1 scallion, finely sliced

1 teaspoon black sesame seeds

Taste of Tomoko (page 266), to taste

In a small bowl, soak the wakame in water for 10 minutes, or until rehydrated. Set aside.

Bring the water to a boil in a medium pot and add the kombu. Remove from the heat, leaving the kombu to steep. After a few minutes, remove the kombu. Set aside about ¼ cup of the steeping water and pour the remaining steeping water back into the pot. Mix the miso into the reserved water and stir to combine. Pour it into the pot along with the wakame, tamari and carrot. Warm the mixture, but do not boil. Add more tamari, to taste, and top with the scallions, sesame seeds and Taste of Tomoko.

SERVES 4

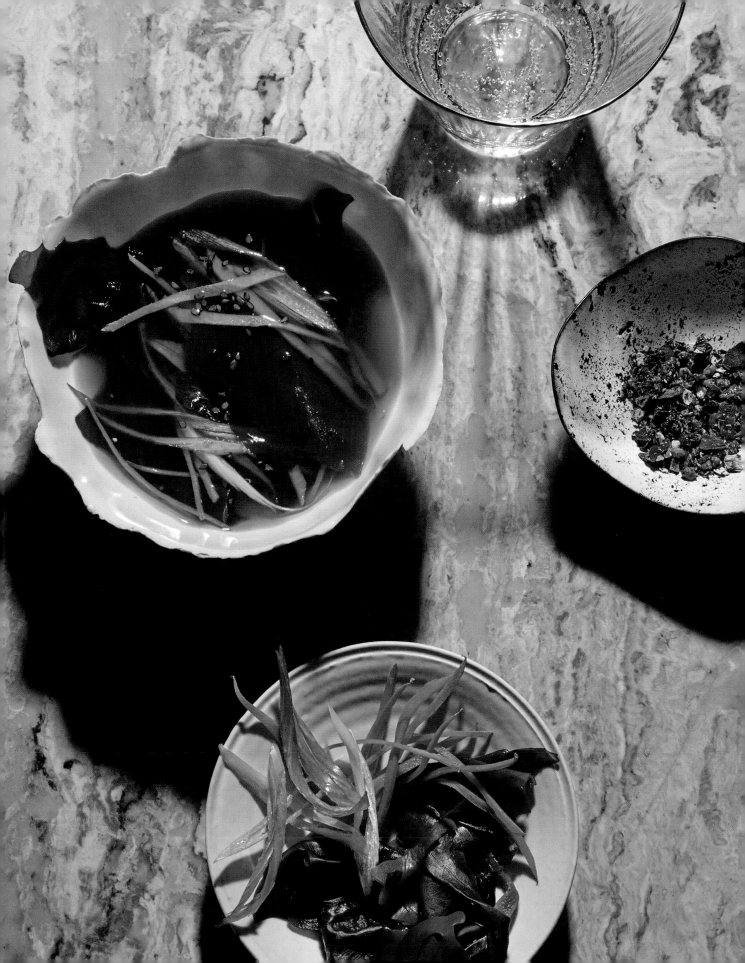

Another *farinata*, like the one in spring (page 46), but this time, it's tailored to the bounty of winter. The classic combination of orange and green adds both sweet and savory and packs this plant-based frittata with color and nutrition. A perfect meal to prepare after a trip to the farmer's market, we like to keep one on hand and pack it to go. Take out never tasted so good.

A WINTER IN DELHI *FARINATA*

1½ cups chickpea flour

2 cups water, vegan bone broth or No Bones about It Broth (page 263)

2 teaspoons curry powder

1¼ teaspoons Himalayan pink salt

4 tablespoons olive or coconut oil

1 large sweet potato, peeled and diced into ½-inch cubes

1 Spanish onion, halved and sliced into ¼-inch rings

2 cups chopped Swiss chard

Soak the chickpea flour with the water or broth, curry powder, ½ teaspoon of the salt and 1 tablespoon of the oil overnight to allow it to ferment, covered so skin doesn't form.

Preheat the oven to 350°F. In a large bowl, toss the potatoes with 1 tablespoon of the oil and remaining ¼ teaspoon of the salt. Place them on a sheet tray, and roast for 30 minutes, or until tender and cooked through. Set aside.

Heat a cast iron or other ovenproof skillet over medium high heat. Add the remaining 2 tablespoons of oil, the onions and the remaining salt. Cook, stirring often, being careful not to burn the onions; turn down the heat, if necessary. Once the onions start to caramelize, add the Swiss chard and 1 tablespoon water. Continue to cook and stir until the Swiss chard begins to wilt. Add the sweet potatoes, distributing them evenly. Then, pour the chickpea batter on top. Cook, without stirring, for about 5 minutes, or until you start to see bubbles coming through the top of the batter and the edges begin to set. Turn off the heat and place the entire pan in the oven to cook for about 10 minutes, or until a knife inserted in the center comes out clean. Carefully remove from oven, let cool for about 10 minutes, then cut into slices and serve.

SERVES 4

When breakfast tastes like dessert, and dessert tastes like breakfast. This adaptogenic oatmeal warms you from the inside out and nourishes you for the colder days of winter. Fortify your immune system with the power of maca and reishi, and soothe your mind with mood lifting cacao. The perfect start to a winter morning.

HIMALAYAN HIGH CACAO OATS

1 cup gluten-free rolled oats

2 cups filtered water

¼ teaspoon Himalayan pink salt

1 tablespoon cacao powder

2 tablespoons dried mulberries

1 tablespoon coconut butter

1 teaspoon raw honey

½ teaspoon maca

½ teaspoon reishi or cordycep mushrooms

TOPPINGS (OPTIONAL)

Cacao nibs

Bee pollen

Honey

Mulberries

Flaky salt

Combine the oats, water and salt in a small saucepan. Set over medium heat and bring to a boil. Reduce to a simmer, and add the cacao and mulberries. Cook for 7 to 10 minutes, or until most of the water has been absorbed. Remove from the heat and stir in the butter, honey, maca and mushrooms. Transfer to bowls, and add toppings, if desired.

SERVES 2

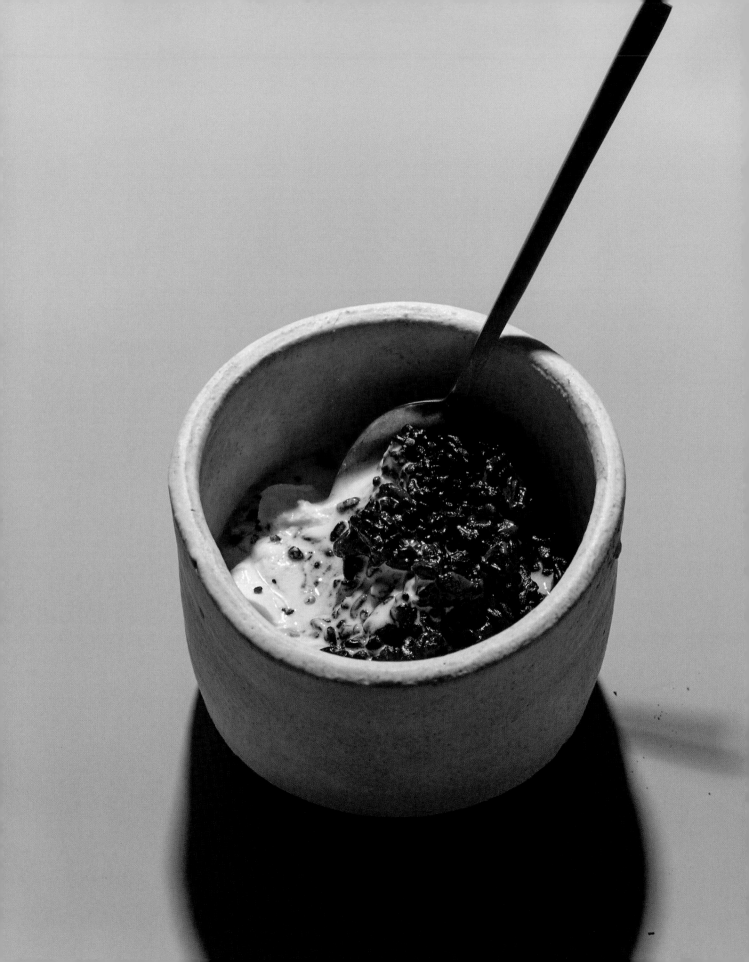

Kerrilynn's husband, John, is the mastermind behind this warming and tropical porridge. With flavors that suggest the East, consider it a breakfast in Bali. Minus the bikini.

FORBIDDEN PORRIDGE

1 cup black rice

½ cup coconut milk

1½ cups coconut water

Grated fresh ginger, to taste

1 cardamom, crushed, black seeds removed

Small handful of goji berries

Big pinch of Himalayan pink salt

Coconut yogurt or coconut butter

Black pepper, to taste

Add the rice, milk, coconut water, ginger and cardamom to large pot and bring to a simmer over medium heat. Cover and cook for 30 minutes, or until done. Take the pot off the heat, add the berries and stir, allowing them to steam in the porridge. Add the salt, coconut yogurt or butter and sprinkle with pepper.

SERVES 4

A raw salad incorporating the deep tastes of winter with the dreamier days of summer, this dish is an elegant and easy meal to have on the table in no time. Ground down with the flavor of cauliflower, and rise up with the taste of citrus. Yin and yang, all around.

WHITE LIGHT SALAD

1 head cauliflower, florets thinly sliced (about 4 cups)

1 small fennel bulb (including fronds), thinly sliced

⅓ cup parsley, chopped

½ cup slivered almonds, toasted and chopped, or ½ cup activated almonds, chopped (see Note)

2 oranges

1 tablespoon minced shallot

2 tablespoons brown rice vinegar

½ teaspoon Himalayan pink salt

½ teaspoon raw honey

¼ cup olive oil

¼ cup currants

Combine the cauliflower, fennel (including fronds), parsley and almonds together in a large bowl. Set aside.

Supreme the oranges (cut into segments without membranes). Reserve the segments. Hold the membrane over a small bowl and squeeze to extract the juice. Add the shallot, vinegar, salt and honey, and combine. Slowly pour in the oil to emulsify. Add the currants and let sit for 10 to 15 minutes, or until they become plump.

Pour the mixture over the cauliflower and mix well. When ready to serve, gently fold in the reserved orange segments.

SERVES 2 TO 4

NOTE: Feel free to substitute any other toasted seed or nut in place of the almonds.

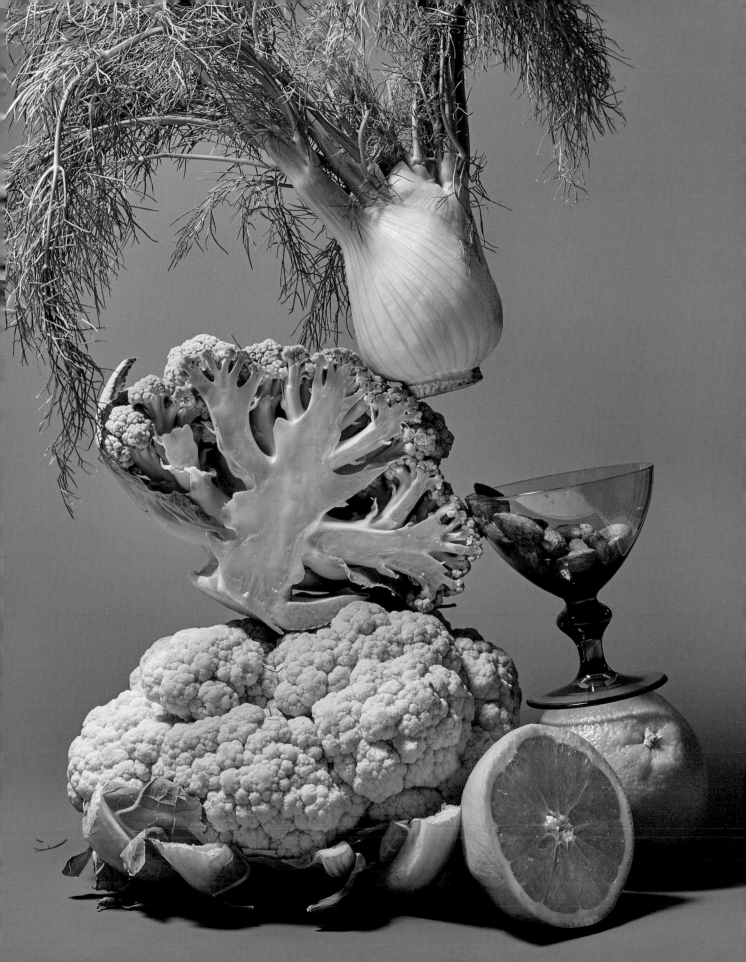

A favorite meal building block of ours, you'll always find a lentil salad in our kitchen. Our version is bright, tart and very French. Just like Cindy's husband, Laurent.

LOVER'S LENTILS

1 cup lentils du puy
or black lentils

2 cups filtered water

1 tablespoon whole-grain mustard

1 tablespoon Dijon
mustard

1 shallot, finely
minced

Large handful of
parsley, chopped, plus
more for garnishing

1 tablespoon apple
cider vinegar

1 tablespoon
Himalayan pink salt,
plus more if needed

2 tablespoons capers,
coarsely chopped

Cherry tomatoes,
halved

Cover the lentils with the water in a large pot, and bring to a boil over medium high heat. Cook for about 20 minutes, or until soft. Don't over-cook them; you want them slightly al dente. Meanwhile, mix together the whole-grain mustard, Dijon mustard, shallot, parsley, vinegar and salt in a large bowl. Drain the lentils, and let cool for a few minutes. Add to the bowl with the vinaigrette, and stir to combine. Top with parsley, capers and tomatoes, and add more salt, if needed. *Bon appétit*!

MAKES 4 SERVINGS

If soup were a cult, this would be its leader. It first gained momentum with Paul Bertolli's version on Food52, and it made waves for its deep and complex flavor, despite its pure simplicity. Gingersnap's Organic in New York City sold a version, and our friend Dana James includes one on her web site, Food Coach NYC. Bertolli's basic recipe needs no improvement, and yet is something of a canvas, allowing it to take new direction. We've boosted ours with turmeric, black pepper and mustard seed for a golden, delicious and thermogenic meal. Yellow mustard seeds will deliver a milder taste, while brown or black mustard seeds are hotter and more pungent. Light your fire, and join the cult.

SOURCE SOUP

2 tablespoons coconut oil

1 yellow onion, chopped

1 (2-inch) piece of turmeric root, grated, or 2 tablespoons dried turmeric

1 teaspoon yellow, brown or black mustard seeds

5 cups filtered water, plus more if needed

1 head cauliflower, chopped into florets

Himalayan pink salt, to taste

Black pepper, to taste

In a Dutch oven or heavy-bottomed soup pan, heat the oil over low heat. Add the onion and turmeric, and cook for 10 minutes, stirring occasionally.

Add the mustard seeds and cook for an additional few minutes. Don't let them burn.

Add 1 cup of the water, turn the heat to medium and bring to a simmer. Then add the cauliflower, cover the pot and let it steam for about 15 minutes.

Add the remaining 4 cups of water, and let simmer, uncovered, for an additional 10 minutes. Blend the soup, using an immersion blender or the Vitamix. Add a big dose of salt and pepper and stir. If the soup is too thick, add some more water.

SERVES 4 TO 6

The vibrant, heady and herby green notes of this curry pair beautifully with the grounding black rice, inviting both heaven and earth onto your plate. Yin and yang at its finest.

GEMINI CURRY BOWL

1 tablespoon coconut oil

3 tablespoons green curry paste

1 (14-ounce) can full-fat coconut milk

3 cups filtered water

2 cups winter squash, cut into ½-inch cubes

1 bird's-eye chili, thinly sliced

1 stalk lemongrass, tough outer layers removed, halved

2 teaspoons fresh turmeric, grated, or 1 teaspoon dried

1 tablespoon fresh ginger, grated

2 small cloves garlic, grated

1 tablespoon coconut aminos or tamari

1 tablespoon fresh lime juice

1½ teaspoons coconut sugar

¼ cup Thai basil or regular basil leaves

1 cup black rice

½ cup unsweetened coconut flakes

½ teaspoon Himalayan pink salt

GARNISHES (OPTIONAL)

Cilantro

Toasted coconut flakes

Toasted slivered almonds

Lime wedges

Place the oil and curry paste in a large sauté pan, and set over medium heat. Cook for 3 to 4 minutes, stirring often. Add the milk and 1 cup of the water, and bring to a boil. Add in the squash, chili, lemongrass, turmeric, ginger, garlic, aminos or tamari, lime juice and sugar. Reduce the heat to a simmer. Cover and cook for 10 to 15 minutes, or until the squash is cooked through. Remove from the heat, discard the lemongrass and stir in the basil. Taste and add more seasoning, if desired.

In another large pan, bring the remaining 2 cups of water to a boil. Stir in the rice, coconut flakes and salt. Reduce the heat to a simmer, and cook for about 15 to 20 minutes, covered, or until most of the liquid has been absorbed. Turn off the heat and keep covered until ready to use.

Fluff the rice and place about ½ cup in the bottom of four shallow bowls. Layer each with 1 cup of the curry, spooning a bit extra of the sauce around the edges of the rice. Top with garnishes (if using).

SERVES 4

Après-ski at its finest. There's nothing we love more than a day at the mountain followed by a meal next to the fire. And, for us, that meal is chili. Spicy, smoky and nuanced, our version includes coffee and cacao, lending an intense and mysterious flavor that we crave.

CHILI COMPLEX

1 tablespoon coconut oil

1 onion, diced

6 cloves garlic, minced

2 tablespoons chili powder

1 teaspoon ground cumin

1 teaspoon ground coriander

½ cup dried lentils, soaked, or 1½ cups cooked

½ cup quinoa

¾ cup grated carrot

¾ cup grated parsnip

1 (28-ounce) can crushed tomatoes

5 cups vegan bone broth, filtered water or No Bones about It Broth (page 263)

½ cup brewed coffee

2 bay leaves

½ bunch thyme or oregano

1 cinnamon stick

1 to 2 tablespoons cacao powder

Himalayan pink salt

GARNISHES (OPTIONAL)

Toasted pumpkin seeds

Lacto-Fermented Hot Sauce (page 256)

Lime wedges

Cilantro

Extra-virgin olive oil

Om Chantilly (page 264)

Heat a large stockpot or Dutch oven over medium heat. Add the oil and the onions, and cook until they become translucent. Stir in the garlic, chili powder, cumin, coriander, lentils, quinoa, carrots and parsnips. Cook for 5 minutes more, stirring often. Add in the tomatoes, broth or water, coffee, bay leaves, thyme or oregano and the cinnamon stick. Raise the heat to high, and bring to a boil. Reduce the heat and gently simmer for at least 2 hours. Remove from the heat when most of the liquid has been absorbed, and the lentils and quinoa are cooked through. Discard the thyme or oregano and the bay leaves. Add the cacao and salt, to taste. Top with garnishes (if using).

SERVES 4 TO 6

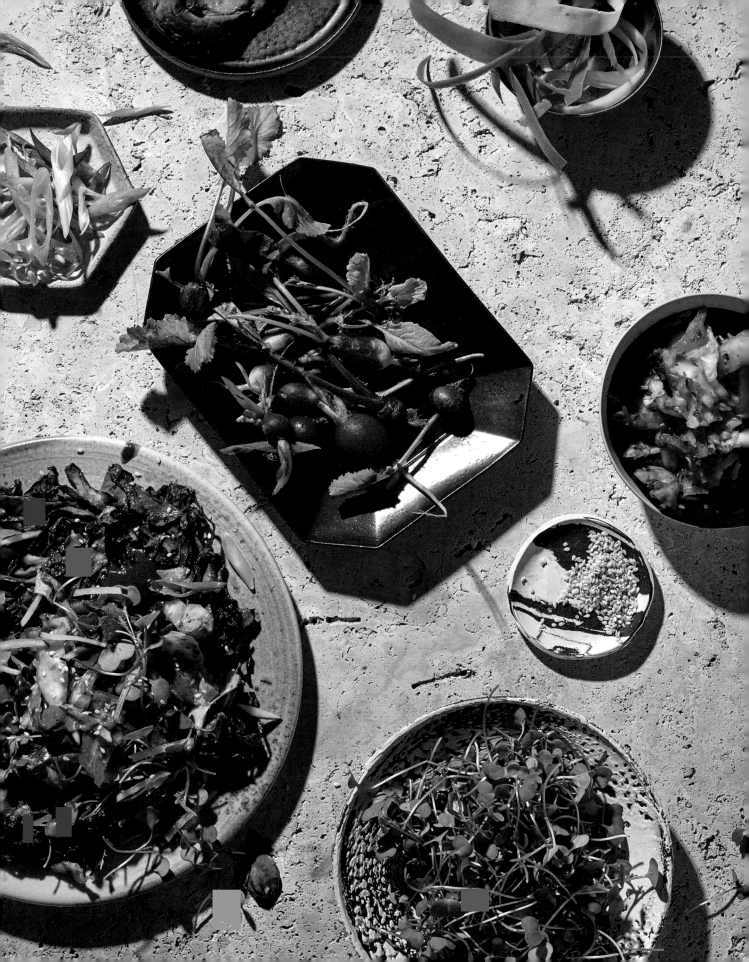

Pancakes inspired by the sea, these fritters spiked with dulse and tamari are a healthy knock-off of Japan's national dish, Okonomiyaki. We top ours with fermented vegetables, scallions, coconut mayonnaise, beet ketchup and schichimi. Let the flavors of the ocean meet the flavors of the East.

DEEP SEA *OKONOMIYAKI*

BATTER

2 cups cabbage, sliced ⅛ inch thick

½ bunch lacinato kale or collard greens, stemmed and sliced ⅛ inch thick

1 large carrot, spiralized or ribboned

1 large parsnip, spiralized or ribboned

1 teaspoon Himalayan pink salt

½ bunch scallions, thinly sliced

½ cup dulse flakes

⅔ cup brown rice flour, plus more as needed

½ cup Aquafaba (page 261)

1 tablespoon tamari

Holy Herbs Schichimi (page 266) or toasted sesame seeds

SAUCE

½ cup coconut mayonnaise

2 tablespoons Bright Right Ketchup (page 261)

1 teaspoon tamari

GARNISHES

Scallions, sliced on the bias

Dulse flakes

Hijiki

Nori powder

Lacto-fermented vegetables

Radishes, julienned

Beets, julienned

Carrots, julienned

Preheat the oven to 350°F.

To make the batter: In a large bowl, mix together the cabbage, greens, carrot, parsnip and salt. Massage well. Transfer to an absorbent kitchen towel and squeeze out any excess moisture. Return them to the mixing bowl. Toss in the scallions and dulse and mix all together. Add in the flour, and toss to coat. Pour in the aquafaba and tamari. Toss once more and allow to rest for 10 to 15 minutes. If the mixture is too wet, add in some more flour, 1 tablespoon at a time.

Using about ¼ cup of the batter, form pancakelike shapes and place them on a parchment-lined baking sheet. Bake for 20 minutes, rotate and bake for an additional 10 to 15 minutes, or until lightly browned and crispy. Remove from the oven and allow to cool slightly.

To make the sauce: In a small bowl, combine the mayonnaise, ketchup and tamari. Set aside.

To assemble: Place each pancake on a serving plate. Drizzle the sauce over top and add any garnishes. Finish with the schichimi or sesame seeds.

MAKES 4 SERVINGS

Bring the islands home. When humble root vegetables are married with spicy jerk seasoning, expect a new kind of roast. Grounding, stabilizing and warming. Get high on the power of Jamaica.

JAMAICAN ROOT ROAST

4 cups root vegetables (turnips, beets, carrots, fennel, onions), chopped into 1-inch cubes

½ teaspoon Himalayan pink salt

1 cup Bless Up Jerk Sauce (page 257)

Scallions, sliced diagonally (optional)

Preheat the oven to 400°F. In a large bowl, combine the vegetables with the salt and jerk sauce. Mix well. Transfer to a parchment-lined baking sheet and bake for 20 minutes, then rotate and roast for another 10 minutes or until cooked through and beginning to caramelize. Serve warm. Add freshly sliced scallions (if using).

SERVES 4 AS A SIDE

France by way of Vietnam. This Southeast Asian take on the French classic, mushroom soup, is as refined as it is deeply satisfying. We could eat this earthy, warming and elegant soup all winter long.

GOLDEN TRIANGLE MUSHROOM SOUP

2 cups Kombu *Dashi* (page 264)

2 teaspoons ginger, grated

Juice of 2 limes

1 (14-ounce) can full-fat coconut milk

1 teaspoon tamari

2 stalks lemongrass, tough outer layers removed, thinly sliced

1 jalapeño, seeded and thinly sliced (wear plastic gloves when handling)

3 cups wild mushrooms (oyster, hen of the woods, shiitake), cleaned

1 tablespoon coconut butter

2 scallions, white and light green parts only, thinly sliced

1 cup cilantro, leaves only

Lime wedges

Place the broth, ginger, lime juice, milk, tamari, lemongrass and jalapeño in a medium saucepan over medium-high heat. Bring to a boil and reduce to a simmer, stirring once to combine. Cook for an additional 5 minutes. Add the mushrooms, and continue to cook for 10 to 15 minutes more, or until the mushrooms are cooked through. Before serving, stir in the butter. Top each bowl with scallions, cilantro and a lime wedge on the side.

SERVES 4

VARIATION

Stir in 1 cup cooked rice noodles, if desired.

When Mexican is in order, we bake a batch of these plant powered enchiladas. A perfectly comforting winter meal, made lighter by their collard green wraps and made delicious by our Three-Seed Mole. This is how we do Mexican. Vegetables, rice and the whole enchilada.

EVOLVED ENCHILADAS

3 cloves garlic, sliced

1 tablespoon olive oil or coconut oil

1 (15 ounce) can pinto beans, rinsed and drained

1 cup cooked brown rice

¼ teaspoon Himalayan pink salt, plus more for cooking water

2 tablespoons fresh lemon juice

1½ cups Three-Seed Mole (page 258)

1 bunch collards, thick stems removed

1 tablespoon sesame seeds

In a deep skillet, sauté the garlic and oil over medium heat until soft. Add the beans, rice, salt and lemon juice, and cook for 5 minutes. Fold in 1 cup of the mole and turn off the heat. Set aside.

Pour 1 to 2 cups of water into a saucepan or skillet that is wide enough to fit a whole flat collard leaf. Make sure you have enough water to fill it 1 inch up the sides of the pan. Add a pinch of salt. Bring to a boil, then reduce the heat to a simmer. Carefully add a few collards at a time. Cook each batch for 1 to 2 minutes, or until bright green. Remove with a slotted spatula onto a paper towel lined plate. Repeat with the remaining collards. Set aside.

Preheat the oven to 350°F. To assemble the enchilada, place ½ cup of the rice and bean mixture horizontally across one end of the collard leaf, leaving at least 1 inch of space on each side. Fold the bottom of the collard over the rice and beans and then tuck in the sides. Continue to tightly roll up the leaf. Transfer to a baking dish, placing the seam side down. Repeat until the tray is completely full. Finally, pour the remaining ½ cup of mole evenly over top the enchiladas and sprinkle with the sesame seeds. Bake for 10 minutes, covered, and for 5 to 10 minutes, uncovered, or until heated through.

SERVES 4

Expect to be surprised by this one. Hiding under the familiarity of "oatmeal," this decadent, transformative and deeply satisfying dish is a welcome change from the expected. Complex and savory, this oatmeal is elevated to a place of sophistication and is ready for even the most refined palate.

DINNER TRANSFORMED

1 or 2 oranges

1 cup gluten-free oats

2 cups filtered water

1½ teaspoons rosemary, minced

1 small garlic clove, microplaned or minced

¼ teaspoon Himalayan pink salt

2 tablespoons botija olives, chopped

2 tablespoons tahini

2 tablespoons toasted pumpkin seeds

1 teaspoon olive oil

Raw honey (optional)

Flaky sea salt

Freshly ground black pepper

Combine the oats, water, rosemary, garlic and Himalayan pink salt in a small saucepan. Set over medium heat, and bring to a boil. Supreme the oranges (cut into segments without membranes). Reserve the segments and the membrane. Reduce to a simmer and stir in the olives. Hold the orange membrane over the pan and squeeze to extract the juice. Cook, stirring often, for 5 to 7 minutes, or until most of the water has been absorbed. Remove from the heat and stir in the tahini. Transfer the mixture into two serving bowls. Top with the pumpkin seeds and reserved orange segments. Drizzle with the oil and honey (if using). Sprinkle with sea salt and pepper.

SERVES 2

Another favorite in our pasta lineup, this healthy take on the classic is a welcome shift. By swapping out pasta noodles for spiralized rutabagas and substituting the traditional cream sauce with an elegant, plant-based version, this dish hits all the right notes. Expect the unexpected.

CAP'S *CACIO E PEPE*

2½ tablespoons olive oil

1 tablespoon chickpea miso

1 tablespoon fresh lemon juice

2 cups rutabaga, spiralized

½ cup Cauliflower Parm (page 251)

Freshly ground black pepper

Salt, to taste

Gently heat the oil in a skillet over low heat. Add the miso and lemon juice, and whisk until emulsified. Add the rutabaga "noodles" and warm through. Remove from heat and transfer to two bowls. Top with the Cauliflower Parm and several cranks of black pepper. Add salt, to taste

SERVES 2

Norwegians do it better. At least according to Kerrilynn's mom. And, since the classic Norwegian gravlax was a favorite of hers from childhood, we set out to create a version that fit into our plant-based world. This unexpected and interesting dish highlights the power of plants and showcases their infinite range. We love plants for so many reasons, and this stunning dish is one of them.

GRAVLAX FOR ZOE

1 large turnip, peeled and sliced ¼ inch thick

¼ cup shredded raw beets

½ cup olive oil, plus more if needed

½ cup grapeseed oil, plus more if needed

1 teaspoon salt

1 teaspoon coconut sugar

½ teaspoon whole allspice

¼ teaspoon caraway seeds

½ teaspoon whole black peppercorns

½ teaspoon mustard seeds

2 tablespoons dulse

4 strips lemon zest

1 teaspoon tamari

5 sprigs of fresh dill

GARNISHES (OPTIONAL)

Capers

Chopped dill

Raw or pickled red onion slices

Lemon wedges

Preheat the oven to 300°F. Place the turnip slices in a single even layer in a deep baking dish. Cover with beets, olive and grapeseed oil, making sure the turnips are submerged. If not, add a bit more oil. Add the remaining ingredients (excluding the optional ingredients), and press down into the oil. Cook for 1 hour. Allow to cool, then refrigerate for 3 hours or overnight. Remove the turnip slices from brine, making sure to brush off any spices. Serve with the capers, dill, onions and lemons (if using).

SERVES 4 TO 6

NOTE: Gravlax cooking oil can be saved and used in vinaigrettes, soups and grain bowls.

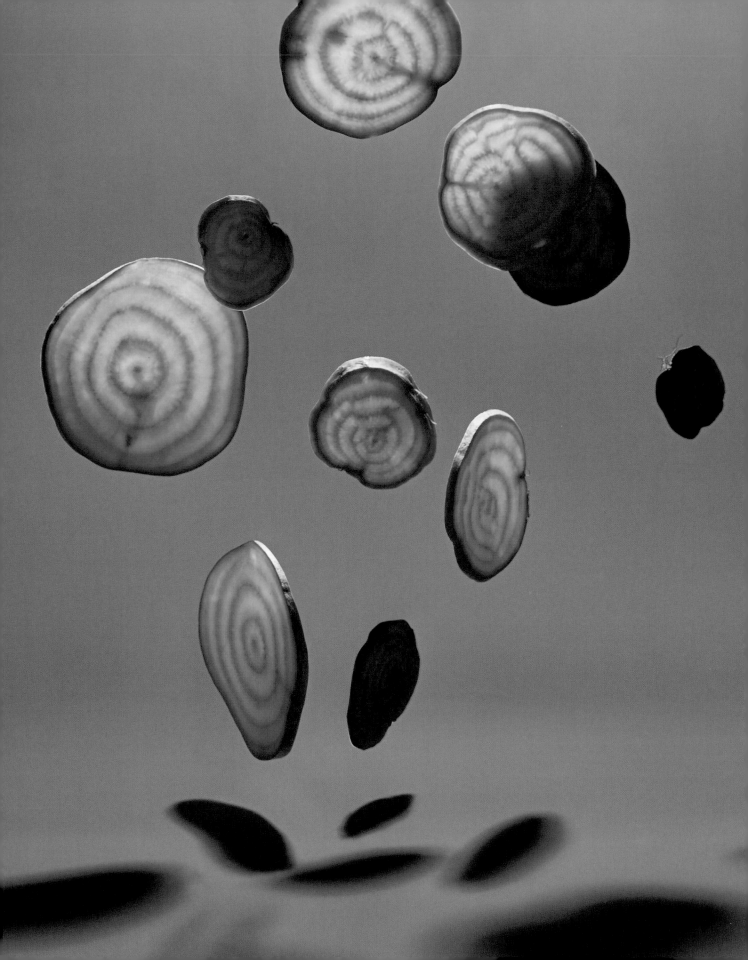

Our version of a salt-and-vinegar chip, but better. These salty, umami snacks are perfect to reach for when the craving hits. Thinly sliced beets marinated with sumac, ume plum vinegar and Himalayan pink salt are an elegant version of one of our favorite treats. Your snack drawer upleveled.

BEACHY BEET CHIPS

4 medium beets, rinsed, scrubbed and tops removed

1 tablespoon olive oil or coconut oil

1 tablespoon sumac

2 tablespoons ume plum vinegar

½ teaspoon Himalayan pink salt

Preheat the oven to 350°F. Slice the beets into $\frac{1}{16}$-inch slices on a mandoline. Place in a large bowl, and add the remaining ingredients. Toss well to combine. Transfer to a few parchment-lined baking sheets in a single layer with no overlapping. Bake for 10 minutes, flip the chips and roast for 5 to 10 minutes more. Chips will crisp as they cool.

Alternatively, you could use a dehydrator set at 125°F for 8 to 12 hours.

SERVES 2

Tea and biscuits go together for good reason. So, we decided to marry the two into one delicious treat. With subtle notes of bergamot from the tea, orange and coconut, this biscotti is elegant and sophisticated. Just like tea time.

TEA-FOR-TWO BISCOTTI

2 cups gluten-free oat flour

1 cup coconut flour

½ cup coconut flakes, toasted

3 tablespoons Earl Grey tea, processed if coarse

½ teaspoon baking powder

¼ teaspoon Himalayan pink salt

1 cup coconut oil

1 teaspoon vanilla extract

Zest of 1 orange

¼ cup fresh orange juice

¾ cup honey

Preheat the oven to 350°F. Combine the dry ingredients in a large mixing bowl. Set aside.

Heat the oil in a small saucepan over low heat until melted, and stir in the vanilla, orange zest, orange juice and honey. Pour over the dry ingredients and mix well. Place the dough on a parchment-lined baking sheet in a rectangular log about 1 inch thick. Bake for 15 minutes, then remove from the oven. Reduce the heat to 250°F. Gently cut the dough log crosswise into 2-inch biscotti pieces. Carefully flip each biscotti on its side and return, then bake for an additional 15 minutes. Allow to cool.

Alternatively, you can dehydrate the biscotti at 125°F for 18 to 24 hours. In this case, slice the dough log into 1-inch biscotti pieces before you put it in the dehydrator.

MAKES 18 TO 24 BISCOTTI

VARIATION

Use chai instead of Earl Grey tea.

Pudding perfection. This sweet treat relies on the abundance of winter pomegranates for a festive dessert worthy of the holidays. Simple yet elegant, it's just right for a dinner party inspired by the season. Merry, merry to you and yours.

VANILLA GEM PUDDING

1 cup seeds or nuts, soaked overnight

1 cup + 2 tablespoons pomegranate juice

1 cup filtered water

1 teaspoon vanilla extract or ½ vanilla bean

¼ cup coconut sugar

¼ teaspoon Himalayan pink salt

1 tablespoon agar-agar flakes

2 teaspoons arrowroot powder

Pomegranate seeds

Bee pollen

Strain the seeds or nuts and transfer them to a high-speed blender. Add in 1 cup of the pomegranate juice and the water. Blend on high for 1 to 2 minutes, or until completely smooth. Strain the mixture through a nut milk bag or cheesecloth. Discard the pulp, or reserve for another use. Place the pomegranate-nut milk into a medium saucepan. Add in the vanilla, sugar, salt and agar-agar. Bring to a boil over medium heat, whisking often. Cover the pan and reduce the heat to a simmer. Continue to simmer for 10 minutes more, stirring every so often, making sure the bottom doesn't burn. In a separate small bowl, combine the remaining 2 tablespoons of pomegranate juice and the arrowroot. Whisk well to combine and slowly add to the saucepan while continuously whisking. Turn up the heat to medium-high. Continue to whisk constantly as the mixture comes to a boil. Remove from the heat and let cool. Transfer to a storage container and refrigerate for at least 2 hours. To serve, scoop the pudding into bowls and top with pomegranate seeds and bee pollen.

SERVES 4

Weeks before her 35th birthday, Cindy found herself on retreat, a yoga retreat that is, in the rolling hills of Tuscany. There, she met some lifelong friends from all over the world who surprised her with not just a birthday cake, but an actual gelato truck. Gelato is the consummate Italian treat, and hazelnuts are a winter favorite. Thanks to a perfect memory, this nutty nice cream will always invoke the power of travel, friendship and, of course, yoga.

BIRTHDAY GELATO

½ **cup hazelnuts**

2 **(14-ounce) cans cold coconut milk**

½ **cup cacao powder**

1 **teaspoon vanilla extract or** ½ **vanilla bean**

¼ **cup maple syrup**

¼ **cup cacao nibs**

Preheat the oven to 350°F.

Place the hazelnuts on a baking sheet and roast for 10 minutes, or until they begin to darken and become aromatic. When cool enough to handle, rub off the skins with a clean kitchen towel. Roughly chop and reserve.

Meanwhile, place a large metal bowl and the corresponding whisk or beater attachment in the freezer for at least 1 hour before preparation. Carefully scoop out the coconut cream from the top of the cans and transfer that into the chilled bowl. Discard the coconut water or reserve it for another use. Begin to whip the cream on high speed, until aerated and soft peaks begin to form. Add in the cacao powder, vanilla and syrup and whip for 1 minute longer. Gently fold in the reserved hazelnuts and the cacao nibs. Remove and place in a small cake pan. Immediately put in the freezer to chill for at least 6 hours. When ready to serve, scoop with an ice cream scoop, and enjoy!

SERVES 4 TO 6

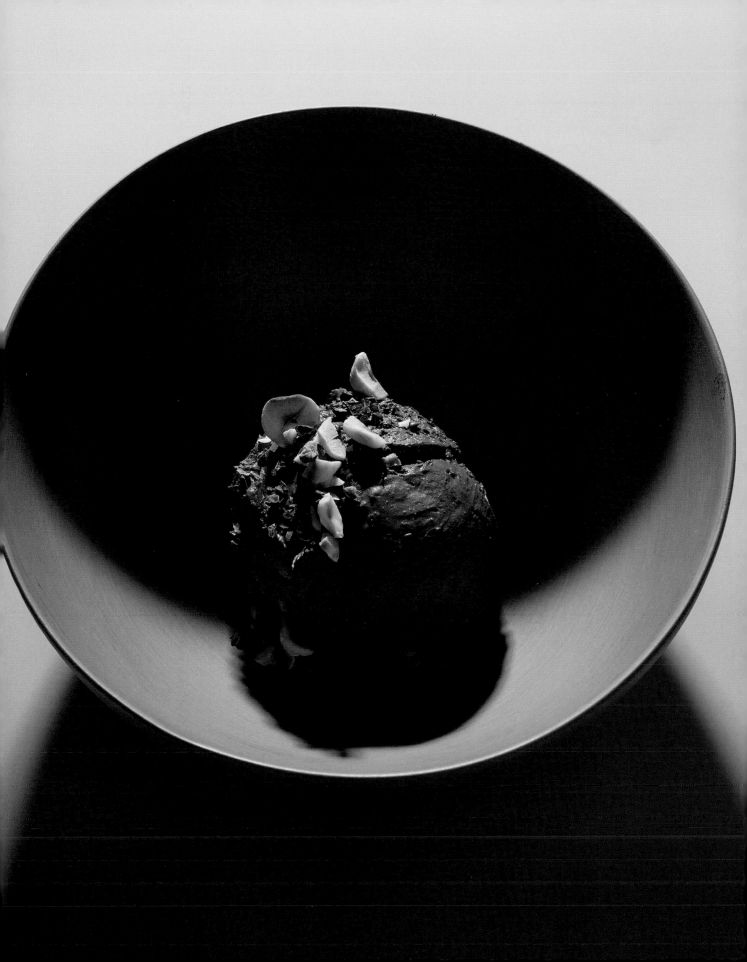

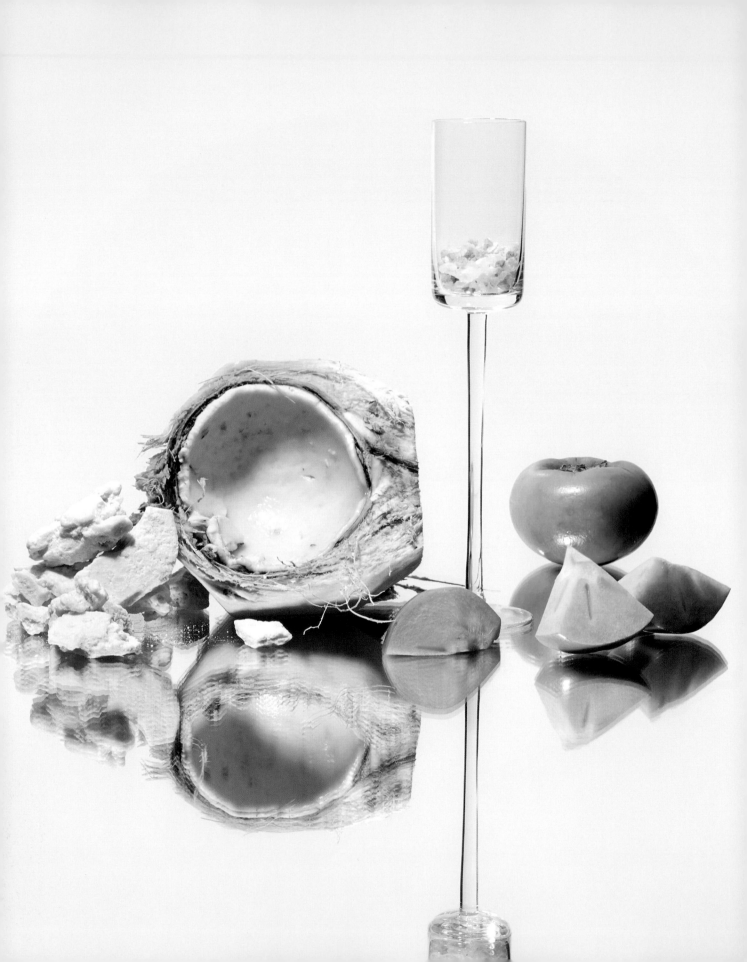

Cindy's mom, Weezie, made a gorgeous holiday cake that was sweetened with ripe fresh persimmons. It was a nod to California and tasted like the sunshine, even in the heart of an East Coast winter. Persimmons are a CAP Beauty favorite, and this holiday bark shines its light.

WEEZIE'S PERSIMMON BARK

2 persimmons, peeled and coarsely chopped

1½ cups raw cacao butter, grated

¾ cup coconut oil

¼ cup coconut sugar

1 teaspoon vanilla extract or ½ teaspoon vanilla powder

2 teaspoons lucuma powder

½ teaspoon Himalayan pink salt (optional)

Place the persimmons in a blender and puree on high until smooth. Set aside.

In a double boiler over medium heat, combine the cacao butter, oil, sugar, vanilla and lucuma. Cook for 3 to 4 minutes, whisking until well-blended and the sugar has dissolved. Pour onto a parchment-lined baking sheet. Spread out in an even, thin layer. Spoon the persimmon puree on top. With a butter knife, drag the puree throughout the white chocolate to create a marble effect. Sprinkle the salt (if using) over the bark. Place the baking sheet into the refrigerator or freezer to chill for 1 hour. Break the bark into pieces and serve.

MAKES ONE 9 X 13-INCH COOKIE SHEET

Set the stage for a good night's sleep with the magic of adaptogenic herbs. Ashwagandha may be India's favorite cure-all but it also does wonders for the stressors of the Western world. Our favorite evening tonics always include this powerfully calming and anti-inflammatory root. The addition of a healthy fat from coconut butter helps to slow down its release for a good night, sleep tight adieu to the day.

SLEEP TIGHT TONIC

½ teaspoon ashwagandha root powder

½ teaspoon ground cinnamon

½ teaspoon ground cardamom

½ tablespoon coconut butter

1 tablespoon tocotrienols

Splash of nut, seed or coconut milk

1 teaspoon of lucuma powder or raw honey (optional)

½ teaspoon vanilla bean powder or ¼ teaspoon vanilla extract (optional)

6 ounces hot water

Pinch of nutmeg

Place all ingredients, except the nutmeg, in a high-speed blender for 1 minute. Pour into your favorite mug, and add the nutmeg.

SERVES 1

Our friend Jamie of the much-loved neighborhood spot, Gingersnap's Organic, introduced us to the power of this drink. Our version incorporates vanilla, a shot of ginger juice, cinnamon and nut milk. We then spike it with adaptogens, depending on the time of day. Mucuna for morning, cordycep mushrooms for afternoon and ashwagandha for evening.

GINGERSNAP'S LATTE

1 cup nut milk

½ teaspoon ground cinnamon

½ teaspoon ashwagandha or other herb

½ teaspoon vanilla extract

½ date

1 tablespoon freshly squeezed ginger juice

In a small saucepan over medium heat, warm the milk and add the cinnamon, ashwagandha, vanilla, date and ginger juice. Add to a high-speed blender and blend on medium for a minute. Strain into your favorite mug and enjoy.

SERVES 1

Our love for Kundalini yoga and its transformative powers knows no bounds. We especially like what it does for our minds and swear by its ability to shift how we feel fast. One of our favorite ways to take the practice off the mat (or the sheepskin) is to brew up a big batch of yogi tea. Spiked with warming herbs that keep us lit from within, we drink it all day. At least when we're not practicing Kundalini.

BHAJAN'S BREW

8 cups filtered water

16 black peppercorns

16 cardamom pods, cracked open

14 cloves

2 cinnamon sticks

8 slices of ginger root, 1" long

3 black tea bags (optional)

2 cups nut or seed milk (optional)

2 tablespoons honey (optional)

Bring the water to a boil in a large pot over medium-high heat. Add the peppercorns, cardamom, cloves, cinnamon sticks and ginger. Cover and boil for 15 minutes. Add the tea (if using) and let steep off the heat for 5 minutes. Remove the tea bags and spices and add in the milk (if using). Do not bring to a boil, when it is just shy of boiling, remove from heat. Sweeten with honey (if using).

SERVES 6 TO 8

We love the Mexican tradition of mixing chocolate with spice. The warming and anti-inflammatory benefits of thermogenic spices meet the radical antioxidant power of cacao, quite possibly our favorite superfood of all. Hot chocolate becomes a health tonic. We'll take two, please.

HOT HOT CHOCOLATE

4 cups homemade nut,
seed or coconut milk

1 small smoked chile
or a pinch of smoked
chile flakes

2 cinnamon sticks,
broken into pieces, or
1 teaspoon ground
cinnamon

1 tablespoon
cardamom pods

2 star anise

½ teaspoon whole
cloves

½ cup cacao powder

1 big spoonful coconut
butter

1 or 2 dates, pitted
and chopped, or
1 teaspoon maple
syrup

Place the milk, chile, cinnamon, cardamom, anise and cloves in a medium saucepan and bring to a simmer over medium heat. Remove from the heat, cover and let stand for 15 minutes. Strain, discarding the spices, and return the milk to the pan. Over medium low heat, whisk in the cacao, butter, and dates or syrup until the chocolate is dissolved and the mixture is warm. Transfer to a high-speed blender, blend and serve in your favorite mugs or bowls.

SERVES 4

NOTE: If using maple syrup, no blending required.

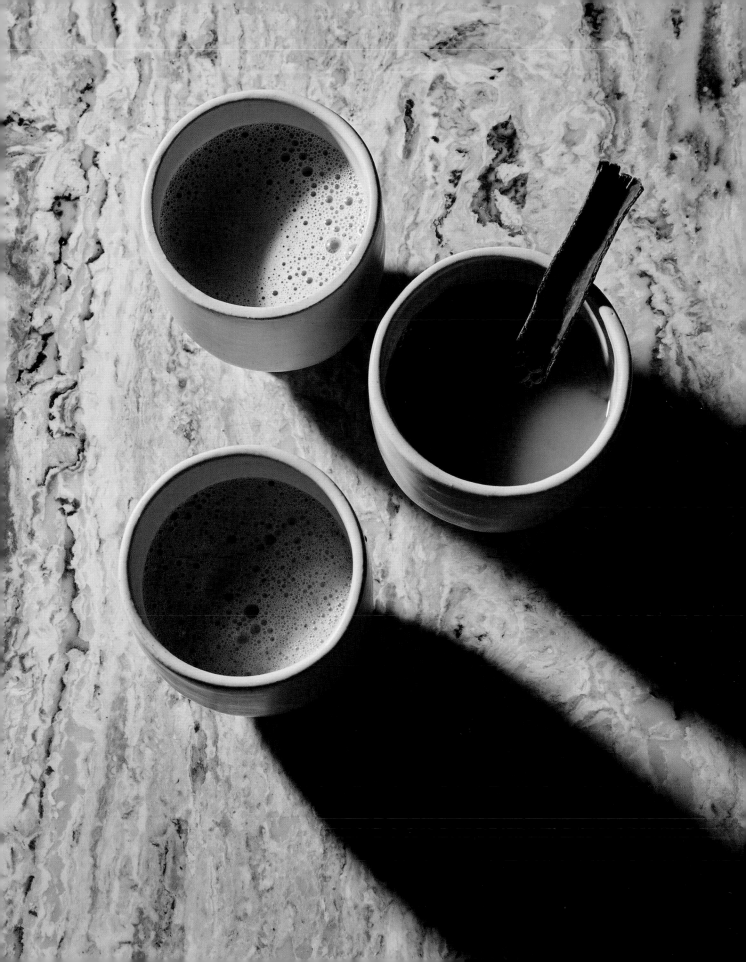

HIGH VIBE STAPLES

The perfect nutrient dense addition to tonics, teas, matcha and smoothies, you can always find a bottle of homemade nut milk in our fridge.

NUT MILK NIRVANA

1 cup raw nuts
(almonds, cashews,
brazil nuts and filberts
all work beautifully)

4 cups filtered water,
plus more for soaking

Splash of vanilla
extract (optional)

⅛ teaspoon salt
(optional)

1 medjool date, pitted
(optional)

1 tablespoon coconut
butter or coconut oil
(optional)

Place the nuts in a large bowl and cover with filtered water. Let soak overnight. Rinse and drain, and add to a high-speed blender. Add the water, vanilla (if using), salt (if using), date (if using) and butter or oil (if using). Blend on high speed for 30 to 60 seconds. Strain through a nut bag and store in the fridge.

MAKES 4 CUPS; SHELF LIFE: 3 TO 5 DAYS

NOTES: Feel free to play with the water ratio, as less water will yield a thicker, more creamlike milk. Combining different types of nuts is great, too, but always make sure that they're activated, in order to enhance their digestibility. If you don't have time to soak the nuts, try a seed milk instead. We love to dehydrate the nuts left over after straining the milk and turn them into flour for a later use. Or, you can add a small amount to a smoothie. Your choice.

Our alternative to nut milk, this seed milk is perfect. We think it's important to diversify, especially when it comes to nuts, and this is a great option. The coconut butter or oil offers antibacterial properties, allowing a longer life in the fridge. Not that you'll need it; you're bound to use this up right away. It's that good.

POWER-UP SEED MILK

1 cup sunflower seeds, pepitas or hemp seeds

4 cups filtered water, plus more for soaking

Splash of vanilla extract

⅛ teaspoon salt (optional)

1 pitted date

1 tablespoon coconut butter or coconut oil (optional)

Place the seeds in a large bowl and cover with filtered water. Let soak overnight. Rinse and drain, and add to a high-speed blender. Add the water, vanilla, salt (if using), date and coconut butter or oil (if using). Blend on high speed for 30 to 60 seconds. Strain through a nut bag and store in the fridge.

MAKES 4 CUPS; SHELF LIFE: 3 TO 5 DAYS

Cheese made from cauliflower. This modern take on nut cheese is lighter than its counterpart and totally delicious. With a savory and umami flavor, this "cheese" is a welcome addition to our fridge. And, we're not nuts.

CAULIFLOWER PARM

2 cups cauliflower florets

1 teaspoon coconut aminos

1 tablespoon olive oil or coconut oil

1 teaspoon fresh lemon juice

⅓ cup nutritional yeast

¼ teaspoon salt

Preheat the oven to 375°F. In a food processor, chop the cauliflower finely until it resembles grains of rice. Transfer to a large bowl and add the aminos, oil, lemon juice, yeast and salt. Combine thoroughly. Place the mixture onto a parchment-lined baking sheet and pat down to create a thin even layer. Bake for 15 minutes, then fluff the "rice," and cook for an additional 15 minutes. Remove from the oven and allow to cool.

Alternatively, you can use a dehydrator set at 125°F for 8 to 12 hours.

MAKES 1 CUP

Our take on the Tex-Mex phenomenon of *queso*, consider this the healthier, friendlier version. Sunflower seeds, nutritional yeast and chickpea miso come together to create a nuanced and delicious alternative to the original version. Because everything's better in Texas.

SUNFLOWER *QUESO*

1 cup sunflower seeds

Filtered water

1 large chopped Spanish onion, chopped

2 small cloves garlic, sliced

1 tablespoon olive oil or coconut oil

2 cups No Bones about It Broth (page 263)

½ teaspoon ground turmeric

½ teaspoon pimenton

1 tablespoon chickpea miso

1 tablespoon tamari

⅓ cup nutritional yeast

Fresh lemon juice, to taste

Salt, to taste

Place the seeds in a large bowl and cover with filtered water. Let soak for 2 hours. Rinse and drain. In a large skillet, sauté the onion and garlic in the oil until they are soft and translucent. Transfer to a high-speed blender. Add the seeds, broth, turmeric, pimenton, miso, tamari and yeast. Blend on high until smooth. Taste and add lemon juice or salt, if desired. Gently warm in a large saucepan over low heat before using.

MAKES 4 CUPS

Cheeses made from activated nuts and seeds help us crowd out dairy and never miss a thing. Creamy sweet cashews are the perfect base for a simple white "cheese" that will stand in perfectly for traditional mild cheeses. Use it for sandwiches or as base for simple herbed dips or dressings. This is one giant step for your plant-based kitchen.

CASHEW QUARK

1½ cups cashews

½ cup filtered water, plus more for soaking

2 probiotic pills

Olive oil, to taste

Himalayan pink salt, to taste

Fresh lemon juice, to taste

Place the cashews in large bowl and cover with filtered water. Let soak for 2 hours or overnight. Rinse and drain, and add them to a food processor with the ½ cup of water. Process until smooth, and similar in texture to ricotta cheese. Open and empty the pills into the cashews and pulse once or twice to combine. Transfer the mixture to a jar with a lid. Place in a dehydrator at 105°F for 8 to 12 hours, or until the desired level of fermentation is achieved. Taste and add oil, salt and lemon juice, to taste.

MAKES 1 CUP

NOTE: To incubate without a dehydrator, wrap the jar in a towel and place it in a turned-off oven (with just the pilot light on) for 12 to 24 hours.

Our version of ricotta relies on the versatility of sunflower seeds, apple-cider vinegar and lemon for its nuanced yet familiar flavor. Perfect as a sweet or savory addition to your meal, this bright staple is a constant in our kitchens. Lighten up.

SUNFLOWER RICOTTA

1 cup sunflower seeds

¼ cup filtered water, plus more as needed and for soaking

1 tablespoon apple cider vinegar

1 tablespoon fresh lemon juice

1 tablespoon nutritional yeast

1 teaspoon Himalayan pink salt

1 tablespoon olive oil or The Daily Hit (page 217)

Place the seeds in large bowl and cover with filtered water. Let soak for 2 hours. Rinse and drain, and add them to a food processor. Add the water, vinegar, lemon juice, yeast, salt and oil, and process until the desired texture is reached. Add more water, if needed. Allow to rest for an hour or so for best flavor. Store in an airtight container.

MAKES 1 CUP; SHELF LIFE: 3 TO 5 DAYS

Passing on dairy shouldn't mean forgoing the tangy and oh-so-versatile taste of full fat yogurt. We use it as the main event, like in a yogurt parfait, or as a garnish to add to dhals, curries and dragon bowls. Coconut yogurt is even more delicious, rich in healthy fats and, like its cousin, is loaded with gut-friendly bacteria. This cooling condiment will fast become a favorite. The variations are endless. Works well as a base for savory applications as well as sweet.

COCONUT YOGURT

2 (15-ounce) cans full-fat coconut milk or 2 cups fresh young coconut meat

1 to 2 teaspoons coconut sugar or maple syrup (optional)

½ cup filtered water or coconut water (optional)

2 probiotic pills or 2 tablespoons store-bought coconut yogurt

If using coconut milk, refrigerate cans overnight. Open them and scoop out the cream into a large saucepan. Discard the coconut liquid (or reserve to use in smoothies, tonics, or when cooking grains or oats). Add the sugar or syrup to the pan now (if using). If using fresh coconut, combine coconut meat and water together in a high-speed blender. Blend until smooth and transfer to a large saucepan.

Gently warm over medium-low heat. Stir often. When the cream reaches 100°F, turn off the heat. Open and empty the probiotic pill or yogurt into the pan, then mix well. Transfer to a quart-size sterilized jar with a lid. Place in a dehydrator away from the heating element. Dehydrate at 105°F for 8 to 12 hours, or until the desired level of fermentation is achieved. Refrigerate for at least 4 hours to set before enjoying.

MAKES 2 CUPS

NOTE: To incubate without a dehydrator, wrap the jar in a towel and place it in an oven (with just the pilot light off) for 12 to 24 hours.

VARIATION

For a thinner, kefir-style yogurt, use the whole can of coconut milk (or more liquid if using fresh meat).

We like to keep this pot full and at the ready for easy lunches, dinners and even breakfasts. An excellent building block for a simple meal, make these on a day when you're at home, knowing you'll have them when you need them. A perfect pot indeed.

PERFECT POT OF BEANS

1 pound beans (we love all of the Rancho Gordo varieties)

1 (6-inch) piece of kombu

Filtered water

1 onion, skin on, quartered, or 1 shallot, sliced

1 head of garlic, halved

3 chile de arbols

1 chipotle pepper

1 tablespoon Himalayan pink salt, plus more if needed

TOPPINGS (OPTIONAL)

Avocado

Cilantro

Coconut yogurt

Place the beans and kombu in large bowl and cover with filtered water. Let soak overnight. Rinse and drain, and add them to a large pot with enough water to cover by a few inches. Add the onion or shallot, garlic, chile, chipotle and salt. Over medium high heat, bring to a hard boil for 10 to 15 minutes. Remove the kombu. Lower the heat and gently simmer, partially covering the pan with a lid. Cook for 1 to 2 hours, checking every $\frac{1}{2}$ hour or so, or until the beans are soft and fully cooked. You might need to add more water, so they don't get too dry. Check for seasonings, as you may need more salt. Remove the chiles, garlic and onion and serve. Add the toppings you like (if using) and enjoy.

MAKES 6 TO 8 SERVINGS (OR 2½ QUARTS)

Some like it hot. We like it fermented. This spicy sauce delivers the best of both worlds. Upgrade your hot sauce, and take the heat.

LACTO-FERMENTED HOT SAUCE

2 cups filtered water

2 tablespoons Himalayan pink salt

4 cups chopped hot or mild peppers, seeded (wear plastic gloves when handling)

4 cloves garlic

2 bay leaves

2 whole cloves

1 teaspoon mustard seeds

1 teaspoon toasted cumin

1 teaspoon whole coriander

Fresh thyme and/or oregano

In a large bowl, whisk together the water with the salt until it dissolves. Set aside.

Pack the peppers, garlic, bay leaves, cloves, mustard seeds, cumin, coriander and thyme and/or oregano into a quart-size jar. Wrapping them in cheesecloth first will make it easier to remove later. Pour the salted water on top, making sure that all the ingredients are submerged in the liquid. You can do this with another small jar or a small plate heavy enough to weigh down the peppers. Seal the jar with the lid. Allow this to ferment at room temperature for at least 3 days, and up to 2 weeks. Open the jar very quickly once daily to release some of the built-up gases. When the peppers reach the desired level of fermentation, drain them, reserving the brine. Transfer the peppers and garlic into a blender. Discard any leftover herbs or spices. Process the peppers until broken down. Add in some of the reserved brine until it reaches the desired consistency. You can also add in brine from other ferments for an interesting flavor contrast (kimchi, sauerkraut, kvass). If you prefer a smoother sauce, pass it through a food mill or fine-mesh sieve. Store the sauce in the refrigerator in a glass jar with lid. It will keep for 1 week.

MAKES 2½ TO 3 CUPS

Heidi Swanson is a goddess in our book. And, one we turn to constantly for inspiration. So, when we happened upon her recipe for black sesame *otsu* (her interpretation of a sesame sauce by way of Japan), we were intrigued. Our version relies on the flavors of Japan and Korea, and it is the perfect condiment to keep on hand in the fridge. Add it to anything that you like. It's good with everything.

BLACK *OTSU*

1 tablespoon toasted sunflower seeds

½ cup toasted black sesame seeds

1 tablespoon hemp seeds

1 teaspoon coconut sugar

1 tablespoon coconut aminos or tamari

2 tablespoons brown rice vinegar

Juice of ½ lemon

1 tablespoon toasted sesame oil or The Daily Hit (page 217)

Using a food processor, spice grinder or mortar and pestle, coarsely grind the sunflower seeds, sesame seeds and hemp seeds. Transfer to a small bowl, add the sugar, aminos or tamari, vinegar, lemon juice and oil, and mix well to combine. Use immediately or refrigerate. Store in an airtight container.

MAKES ABOUT ½ CUP

Turn up the heat, CAP Beauty style. This sauce takes grilled or roasted veggies to the Islands and back. Fire up the grill. Deliver us to paradise.

BLESS UP JERK SAUCE

½ cup chopped mango

3 tablespoons fresh lime juice

2 scallions, white and light green parts only, chopped

2 scotch bonnet or habanero peppers, seeded and chopped (wear plastic gloves when handling)

3 cloves garlic

2 tablespoons fresh thyme, de-stemmed

1 tablespoon grated fresh ginger

2 tablespoons brown rice vinegar

1 teaspoon ground allspice

1½ teaspoons coconut sugar

2 teaspoons Himalayan pink salt

⅓ cup olive oil

Combine all ingredients in a high-speed blender and puree until smooth. Keep refrigerated. Store in an airtight container.

MAKES 1 CUP

Our version of a threesome. Pumpkin seeds, sunflower seeds and sesame seeds come together to spread the love. This complex yet grounding sauce is a favorite of ours, and one we turn to often. We love it in a taco, as a base for a salad dressing or for making Evolved Enchiladas (see page 234). Use it up; it's not complicated.

THREE-SEED MOLE

3 dried ancho or guajillo chiles (wear plastic gloves when handling)

¾ cup pumpkin seeds

½ cup sunflower seeds

2 tablespoons sesame seeds

½ yellow Spanish onion, halved and sliced in ¼-inch half-moons

1 tablespoon coconut oil

½ tablespoon Himalayan pink salt, plus more if needed

1 teaspoon ground cumin

1 teaspoon dried oregano

1 tablespoon tomato paste

1 tablespoon currants

1½ cups unsalted vegetable stock

1 tablespoon cacao powder

½ teaspoon cinnamon

1 teaspoon coconut aminos

1 tablespoon fresh lemon juice

Wearing plastic gloves, remove the seeds from the chiles. Bring 2 cups water to a boil and add the chiles. Soak for 30 minutes.

Using the same skillet over medium high heat, cook the pumpkin seeds for 2 to 3 minutes, or until they begin to pop. Shake the skillet often, so they do not burn. Remove and set aside. Proceed with the sunflower seeds, and then the sesame seeds. It is important to cook each type of seed separately, as they all have different toasting times. Transfer all the toasted seeds to a food processor and process until finely ground. Set aside.

In a heavy-bottomed saucepan over medium heat, sauté the onions in the oil and salt until they are soft and translucent. Reduce the heat to medium low and add in the cumin, oregano, tomato paste and currants. Cook, stirring often, for about 3 minutes, or until the tomato paste begins to darken. Then, add in the stock, the reserved chiles and the reserved seeds, and bring to a boil. Reduce to a simmer and gently cook for about 10 minutes longer. Remove from the heat and stir in the cacao, cinnamon, aminos and lemon juice. Transfer mixture to a blender, and puree well. (Be very careful, as the mole will still be very hot). Season, to taste, with more salt, if desired. Store in an airtight container.

MAKES 2 CUPS

A batch of this spread made from raw botija olives adds salt, healthy fat and big time flavor to crudités. We take the cultural mashup a step further, and spike it with a touch of Japanese nori for a very nontraditional interpretation of a South of France classic. Especially delicious with fennel, carrots and watermelon radishes. *Oisshi, Buen Provecho* and *Bon Appétit!*

BLACK MAGIC TAPENADE

1 small garlic clove, chopped

2 sheets nori

½ cup botija olives, pitted

½ cup Castelvetrano olives, pitted

2 tablespoons fresh lemon juice

½ cup olive oil

½ bunch of parsley, leaves only

Combine the garlic, nori, olives, lemon juice and oil in a food processor, and process until well-combined. Add in the parsley leaves and pulse a few times to incorporate. Serve with crudités or use as a spread. Store in an airtight container.

MAKES ABOUT 1 CUP

A classic relish adds bite and flavor to sandwiches and salads. Ours is (big surprise!) fermented.

RELISH THE RELISH

3 cups shredded kirby cucumbers

1 shallot, diced

1 teaspoon dill seeds or ½ bunch dill

½ teaspoon turmeric

½ teaspoon black peppercorns

2 tablespoons Himalayan pink salt

Filtered water, if needed

Combine the cucumbers, shallot, dill, turmeric, peppercorns and salt into a large bowl. Massage the ingredients together to marry the flavors. Transfer to a 1-quart jar, pressing down firmly after each addition. You want the relish to be submerged underneath the liquid. If necessary, add the water, 1 tablespoon at a time. Cover tightly and allow to sit at room temperature for 2 to 5 days, or until the desired level of fermentation is achieved. Will keep for 1 month in the refrigerator.

MAKES ABOUT 2 CUPS

Thanks to his uncle Klaas, Cindy's son, Louis, is a mayonnaise-lover. A one-time apprentice of Daniel Bouloud and a good Belgian son, Klaas makes his mayonnaise with fresh raw eggs. We turn instead to aquafaba, the mysterious and magical cooking liquid from chickpeas. We love this plant-based mayo on a big raw veggie sandwich. Klaas and Louis may not approve, but then again, they might not know the difference.

COCONUT MAYONNAISE

¼ cup Aquafaba (opposite)

1 tablespoon fresh lemon juice

1 teaspoon Dijon mustard

¼ teaspoon Himalayan pink salt

½ cup grapeseed oil

½ cup coconut oil, melted

Freshly ground black pepper, to taste

Place the aquafaba, lemon juice, Dijon and salt in a food processor. Process for 15 seconds. Combine the oils, and very slowly drizzle them into the aquafaba mixture while the processor/blender is running. This should emulsify the mayonnaise. Add the pepper, to taste. Transfer to a jar and keep refrigerated.

MAKES 1 CUP

VARIATIONS

Add turmeric for a golden mayo and chopped herbs and avocado for a green goddess mayo. Try roasted garlic for an aioli. Pimenton makes for a smoky Spanish mayo.

With their natural sweetness and vibrant hue, beets make the perfect base for a new-age ketchup. Use it as you would the classic version on potatoes or veggie burgers, or try it on our favorite deep-sea inspired Japanese pancakes. Hot pink is the new red. And, salty-sweet never goes out of style.

BRIGHT RIGHT KETCHUP

2 to 3 beets

6 dates, chopped

½ yellow Spanish onion, chopped (½ cup)

¾ cup apple cider vinegar

1 garlic clove, chopped

1 teaspoon coconut aminos

¼ teaspoon allspice

½ teaspoon Himalayan pink salt

1 teaspoon ground coriander

Preheat the oven to 400°F. Tightly wrap the beets in foil or parchment paper and roast for 45 minutes to 1 hour, or until a knife pierces through them easily. Cool, then peel and chop (you should have about 3 cups).

In a high-speed blender, combine the beets with all the remaining ingredients and puree until completely smooth. Will keep refrigerated for 1 week.

MAKES 2 TO 3 CUPS

The alchemical cooking liquid from chickpeas magically transforms foods and mimics an egg white, allowing us to go where no plant-based chef (or pastry chef) has gone before. Simple, yet complex.

AQUAFABA

1 cup dried chickpeas

Filtered water

Rinse the chickpeas, removing any stones or debris. Place in a large bowl and cover with a few inches of water. Remove any chickpeas that float. Refrigerate and soak for at least 12 hours.

Strain the chickpeas and rinse. Place in a medium pot and cover with water by 2 to 3 inches. Bring to a boil, then reduce to a simmer. Cook for 1 to 1½ hours, or until the chickpeas are tender. Carefully strain the chickpeas and reserve the cooking liquid. Store the chickpeas for another use. Allow the liquid to cool, and then refrigerate. Store in an airtight container.

MAKES 1 QUART

The Europhile's breakfast favorite graces everything from toast to crepes to big slices of raw banana. But, of course, the highly processed store-bought kind falls squarely outside our definition of High Vibrational. But, at its core, we find that hazelnuts and cacao are two whole food ingredients that we can get behind. This makeover is a no-brainer, a long overdue upgrade to a European classic. Keep a jar of this on hand and go continental, CAP Beauty style.

HIGH VIBE HAZELNUT SPREAD

1 cup hazelnuts

½ cup hemp seeds

Coconut oil, as needed

½ cup raw cacao powder

2 tablespoons maple syrup

1 teaspoon vanilla extract or ½ vanilla bean

½ teaspoon Himalayan pink salt

1 teaspoon cordycep mushrooms

Preheat the oven to 375°F.

Place the hazelnuts on a parchment-lined baking sheet. Bake for 10 to 15 minutes, or until toasted and fragrant. Remove from the oven and let cool. Transfer them onto a kitchen towel, and rub off the skins.

Place the nuts and the hemp seeds in a food processor or high-speed blender. Process them until they reach a butter-like consistency, making sure to scrape down the sides often. This may take 8 to 10 minutes. Add in a little coconut oil if they are having trouble breaking down. Add in the cacao, syrup, vanilla, salt and cordyceps, and process until well combined. Store in the refrigerator in an airtight container.

MAKES 1 CUP; SHELF LIFE: 3 TO 5 DAYS

NOTE: You can omit roasting the hazelnuts for a raw version, keeping the nutrient-rich skins on the nuts.

Bone broth has taken the health food world by storm. Since we shy away from bones, we set out to create a CAP Beauty version. Rich with seaweed, vegetables and mushrooms, ours is mineral heavy, highly nutritious and tastes like the sea. Ain't no bones about it.

NO BONES ABOUT IT BROTH

3 (2-inch) pieces of kombu

8 cups filtered water

1 yellow onion, chopped

1 tablespoon olive oil or coconut oil

1 carrot, chopped (about 1 cup)

1 leek, chopped (about 1 cup)

½ cup dried shiitakes or 1½ cups fresh

1 (2-inch) piece of ginger, chopped

1 (2-inch) piece of turmeric root, chopped

1 head garlic, unpeeled, halved crosswise

⅔ cup dulse

8 sprigs of parsley

6 sprigs of thyme

2 bay leaves

1 teaspoon black peppercorns

1 to 2 whole chiles (optional)

In a large pot, soak the kombu in 4 cups of the water overnight.

In a large stockpot, sauté the onions in the oil until they become translucent. Add in the carrot and leek. Continue to sauté for 8 to 10 minutes, or until both vegetables become fragrant and soften.

Add the kombu and its water to the pot. Pour in the remaining 4 cups of water, mushrooms, ginger, turmeric, garlic, dulse, parsley, thyme, bay leaves, peppercorns and chiles (if using). Heat over medium heat. Right before the pot boils, pull out the kombu and discard it. Bring the remaining broth to a boil, then reduce to a simmer. Gently cook, undisturbed, for 2 hours.

Strain the broth carefully through a fine mesh sieve and/or cheesecloth. Discard the vegetables (or save for another use). Taste the broth and add salt, lemon juice, raw cider vinegar or your choice of oil to taste, if desired.

MAKES 1 QUART

VARIATION

Add 1 to 2 teaspoons chlorella or spirulina for an extra sea mineral kick. Make sure to add it after the broth has cooled slightly.

A staple of Japanese food, *dashi* is one of the fastest ways to get a nourishing and delicious dinner on the table. Keep this stock in the fridge or freezer, and mix it up with miso, seaweed, vegetables and buckwheat noodles for a healthy-and-quick meal. We also like to keep it in ice-cube trays for a quick single serving of miso soup. *Oishii!*

KOMBU *DASHI*

2 (2-inch) pieces of kombu

1 (2-inch) piece of ginger, peeled

2 tablespoons dulse

4 cups filtered water

1 teaspoon reishi, cordycep mushrooms or chaga (optional)

In a medium saucepan, bring the kombu, ginger, dulse and water almost to a full boil. Right before it boils, turn off the heat and steep for 15 minutes. Strain, reserving the cooking liquid.

Stir in the mushrooms (if using) when the soup cools a bit.

MAKES 4 CUPS

The French call it chantilly. That's pronounced "Shanti," and we think this may be more than a coincidence. Nothing delivers bliss like an airy and lightly sweet coconut whipped cream. Here's how we do Om Chantilly.

OM CHANTILLY

1 (15-ounce) can full-fat coconut milk

½ teaspoon vanilla extract or ¼ vanilla bean

1 tablespoon liquid sweetener (optional)

Place the unopened can of coconut milk in the refrigerator at least 12 hours.

Place the mixing bowl and whisk/beater attachment in the freezer at least 1 hour before making the whipped cream.

Remove the can of coconut milk from the refrigerator without shaking it. Carefully scoop out the coconut cream from the can and transfer it into the chilled bowl. (Discard the coconut water or reserve it for another use.) Whip the cream on high, until soft peaks form. Add in the vanilla and sweetener, until desired consistency is reached. Use immediately. Whipped cream will harden in the refrigerator.

MAKES 1½ CUPS

Our friend and acupuncturist, Frances, introduced us to this exotic and elegant shake that transforms simply everything. Use it liberally to uplevel any meal, from soups and stews to roast veggies and salads.

NEFERTITI SPICE SHAKE

½ cup pistachios

¼ cup pumpkin seeds

2 teaspoons cumin seeds

2 teaspoons coriander seeds

1 teaspoon fennel seeds

Pinch Himalayan pink salt

1 teaspoon ground sumac

Heat the oven to 350°F. Spread the nuts on a parchment-lined baking sheet. Bake, shaking the pan from time to time, for about 9 minutes, or until the nuts smell sweet and fragrant. Keep a close eye on the nuts to prevent burning. Remove from the oven and let cool completely. Coarsely chop and set aside. Set a small skillet over medium heat. Add the pumpkin seeds and toast for a few minutes, just until fragrant. Remove from the heat, cool completely, and coarsely chop. Return the skillet to the heat. Add the cumin, coriander and fennel seeds to the skillet. Reduce the heat and toast, shaking skillet, for about 1 minute, or until fragrant. Remove from the heat and cool completely. Transfer the spices to a mortar and pestle and crush to a medium to fine texture. Combine the cooled nuts, pumpkin seeds, ground spices, salt and sumac in an airtight container. Shake to combine and enjoy.

MAKES ½ CUP

Schichimi is one of our favorite Japanese blends. Sold near temples since the 17th century, we rely on its umami flavors of citrus, sesame and hemp seeds, chiles, ginger and nori to bring Japan closer. Holy herbs, indeed.

HOLY HERBS SCHICHIMI

Zest of 2 oranges or tangerines

1 tablespoon hemp seeds

2 sheets nori, torn into small pieces

1 teaspoon ground ginger

½ aleppo pepper

1 tablespoon toasted black sesame seeds

1 tablespoon toasted white sesame seeds

Place the orange zest in a dehydrator set at 125°F and dehydrate for 8 to 12 hours, or until sufficiently dried out.

In a high-speed blender, combine the orange zest, hemp seeds, nori, ginger and pepper, and process until finely ground. Add in the sesame seeds, and quickly pulse once or twice to incorporate.

MAKES ½ CUP

When Kerrilynn was a kid, she went through a heavy Japanophile phase. She ate with chopsticks, she wore a kimono, and she went by the name Tomoko. This spice blend is a love letter to all that we love about Japan. Sprinkle it on everything, and bring Japan home (kimono not included).

TASTE OF TOMOKO

6 shiitake mushrooms

3 plum tomatoes, seeded

4 (6 inches each) pieces of kombu

1 tablespoon toasted sesame seeds

2 tablespoons hojicha or genmaicha tea leaves

1 tablespoon dulse

1 teaspoon chili flakes

Place a single layer of mushrooms and tomatoes in an oven set at the lowest setting for 6 hours or a dehydrator set at 125°F for 12 to 18 hours, or until they are sufficiently dried out.

In a food processor, combine all ingredients and blend until finely ground. Store in a glass container for 1 month.

MAKES ABOUT 1 CUP

If Injera (page 270) is the MVP of Ethiopian cuisine, berbere gets the assist. This essential smoky spice blend makes beans and veggies come to life, delivering the warmth and fire of our favorite African food. Keep a jar on hand, and infuse your meals with heat on repeat.

BERBERE

1 tablespoon whole coriander seeds

1 tablespoon whole cumin seeds

5 whole cloves

2 teaspoons whole allspice berries

1 tablespoon smoked paprika

1 teaspoon cinnamon

1 teaspoon cardamom

1 teaspoon turmeric

½ teaspoon ground ginger

½ teaspoon cayenne

½ teaspoon grated nutmeg

½ teaspoon freshly ground black pepper

Place a skillet over medium high heat. Working spice by spice (one at a time), toast the coriander, cumin, cloves and allspice berries. (They will all have different toasting times.) When each spice becomes fragrant and begins to pop, remove it from the pan and set aside. Once the first four spices are complete, place them in a spice grinder or mortar and pestle. Process until finely ground. Remove and place into a mixing bowl along with the remaining ingredients. Stir well to combine. Place in an airtight container for up to 2 weeks, or use immediately.

MAKES ½ CUP

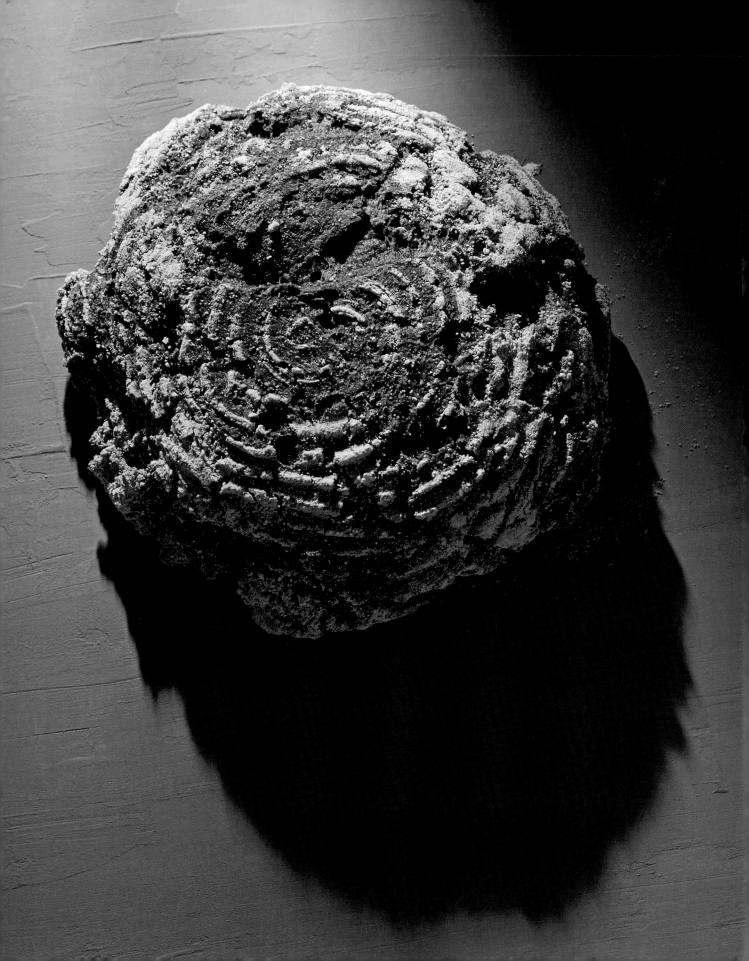

Our take on the classic sourdough. Mesquite, sorghum, oat, millet and buckwheat bake together Dutch oven–style, for a loaf that takes you to San Francisco.

A SOUR BROWN BREAD

STARTER

½ cup sorghum flour

½ cup filtered (dechlorinated) water

1 tablespoon gluten-free sourdough starter/rejuvelac or water kefir

BREAD

4 tablespoons ground flaxseeds

2¼ cups filtered water

2 cups starter

1 cup tapioca starch

1 cup buckwheat flour

1 cup oat flour

1 cup millet flour

½ cup mesquite flour

1 tablespoon Himalayan pink salt

2 tablespoons xanthan gum

¼ cup coconut oil, melted, or olive oil

1 to 2 tablespoons honey or maple syrup

Whisk all starter ingredients in a large bowl to combine. Cover with cheesecloth or a clean kitchen towel, and let rest on the countertop, stirring a few times occasionally, for 8 hours. Add in:

½ cup sorghum flour

½ cup filtered (dechlorinated) water

Whisk again to combine. Continue this pattern switching between sorghum and water for 48 hours. Make sure to whisk a few times between each "feeding." Keep covered. You will start to see bubbling after about 48 hours. At this point, you can start feeding it just once per day. If the starter gets too large, remove ½ cup to 1 cup before adding in fresh flour.

Your starter may take different times, depending on how warm or cold your kitchen is. Once you have at least 2 cups of starter, you can make this bread.

In a small bowl, mix together the flax and 1¼ cups of the water. Let sit until a gel forms. Then add it to a large bowl along with the starter and the remaining 1 cup of water. Mix well and set aside. In a large bowl, combine the tapioca, the flours, salt and xanthan gum. Add the oil and honey or syrup, and mix well. Then slowly, in batches, add the flax mixture, gently massaging together with your hands. Let rest on the countertop for about 8 hours, covered with plastic wrap. Remove about one third of the dough (transfer the rest to the refrigerator for another time) and gently place it on a piece of parchment paper over a flat surface. Allow to rest for about 6 more hours at room temperature. Preheat the oven to 500°F and set an empty Dutch oven inside for at least 30 minutes. Remove with oven mitts and carefully place the sourdough inside using the parchment for easy transfer and removal later. You don't want to agitate the dough too much in this process; it will disrupt the natural sour fermentation. Use a knife to make a few slices on the top of the dough. Place the lid on the pan and bake for about 15 minutes. Remove the lid and continue to bake for an additional 15 to 20 minutes, or until golden brown and crispy. Remove from the oven and allow to cool for 20 to 30 minutes before removing the bread from the Dutch oven.

YIELDS 1 ROUND BOULE OF SOURDOUGH PLUS 2 BACKUPS

We love Ethiopian food. And injera, the staple of any Ethiopian meal, is a favorite. This tart, sour bread takes the place of silverware, and is the perfect way to enjoy the deeply spiced, plant heavy and intoxicating flavors of this exotic cuisine. Try it as a wrap, or add it to a salad. The options are endless. Get creative and use it up.

INJERA

1½ cups teff flour

2 cups filtered water

½ teaspoon Himalayan pink salt

Coconut oil

Combine the flour with the water in a medium bowl. Whisk until well combined. Cover with a clean kitchen towel and let sit at room temperature for 1 to 3 days. The injera batter should begin to bubble and ferment. (Leaving it out longer will result in a more sour flavor.) Whisk the salt into the flour mixture. Heat up a medium nonstick skillet over medium heat. Add a small amount of oil to the pan and heat until the oil is shimmering. Pour about ¼ cup of the batter into the pan. Rotate the skillet so that the batter covers and forms an even layer. Allow to cook until bubbles begin to form around the edges and the bottom starts to naturally release. Remove from the pan and allow to rest. Continue with the remaining batter. Separate the injera with sheets of parchment paper so they do not stick together.

MAKES 8 TO 12

Oats, seeds and faraway spices come together to make the perfect cracker. Dense and savory, consider these your new go to for the cheese board.

SO-MANY-SEEDS CRACKERS

1 cup gluten-free oats, coarsely ground

¼ cup psyllium husks

½ cup pumpkin seeds

½ cup sunflower seeds

¼ cup chia seeds

¼ cup flaxseeds

¼ cup sesame seeds

1 tablespoon nigella seeds (black cumin)

1 clove garlic, grated

2 tablespoons Taste of Tomoko (page 266)

1 tablespoon nori powder

⅓ cup coconut aminos or tamari

2 tablespoons CBD, olive or coconut oil

2 tablespoon fresh lemon juice

2 tablespoons filtered water

½ teaspoon Himalayan pink salt

¼ cup nutritional yeast (optional)

In a large bowl, combine the oats, psyllium husks and all the seeds. Set aside.

In a medium bowl, whisk together all the remaining ingredients. Pour this over the seed mixture and combine thoroughly. Spread out on parchment-lined dehydrator sheets and dehydrate at 115°F for 24 to 36 hours, or until crispy. Break into pieces and enjoy.

MAKES 2 BAKING SHEETS. CRACKER AMOUNT WILL VARY DEPENDING ON YOUR PREFERRED SIZE.

VARIATION

You can roast the crackers in the oven at 300°F for 30 to 45 minutes instead of dehydrating. You can change up the seed ratios, using whatever amounts of each you desire. Just make sure there are about 2 cups of seeds total.

THE RESOURCES

EATING OUT

A guide to our favorite spots for any kind of meal. Some are a quick and fast affair, some warrant staying awhile. These are the places serving up the kind of food we love. Health, wellness and vitality that tastes delicious.

NEW YORK CITY

EL REY COFFEE BAR & LUNCHEONETTE
100 Stanton Street
New York, NY 10002
212-260-3950
elreynyc.com

CAFE CLOVER
10 Downing Street
New York, NY 10014
212-675-4350
cafeclovernyc.com

EN JAPANESE BRASSERIE
435 Hudson Street
New York, NY 10014
212-647-9196
enjb.com

DIMES
49 Canal Street
New York, NY 10002
212-925-1300
dimesnyc.com

SOUEN
210 6th Avenue
New York, NY 10014
212-807-7421
souen.net

INDAY
1133 Broadway
New York, NY 10010
917-521-5012
indaynyc.com

DE MARIA
19 Kenmore Street
New York, NY 10012
212-966-3058
demarianyc.com

THE FAT RADISH
17 Orchard Street
New York, NY 10002
212-300-4053
thefatradishnyc.com

INJERA
11 Abingdon Square
New York, NY 10014
212-206-9330
injeranyc.com

HU KITCHEN
downtown:
78 Fifth Avenue
New York, NY 10011
212-510-8919
uptown:
1536 Third Avenue
New York, NY 10128
212-335-2105
hukitchen.com

JUICE PRESS
212-777-0034
juicepress.com

TWO HANDS RESTAURANT & BAR
251 Church Street
New York, NY 10013
twohandsnyc.com

SWEETGREEN
226 Bleecker Street
New York, NY 10014
917-639-3212
sweetgreen.com

HANGAWI
12 East 32nd Street
New York, NY 10016
212-213-0077
hangawirestaurant.com

THE SHANTI SHACK
85 North 3rd Street
Brooklyn, NY 11249
347-463-9886
shantishack.com

ABC KITCHEN
35 East 18th Street
New York, NY 10003
212-475-5829
abckitchennyc.com

ABCV
38 East 19th Street
New York, NY 10003
212-475-5829
abchome.com/eat/abcv/

QUARTINO
11 Bleecker Street
New York, NY 10012
212-529-5133
quartino.com

MELVIN'S JUICE BOX AT MISS LILY'S
130 West Houston Street
New York, NY 10012
646-588-5375
misslilys.com/melvins-juice/

BRODO BROTH COMPANY
West Village:
496 Hudson Street
New York, NY 10014
212-366-0600
East Village:
200 First Avenue
New York, NY
646-602-1300
brodo.com

TÉ
163 West 10th Street
New York, NY 10014
929-335-3168
te-nyc.com

LOS ANGELES

CAFE GRATITUDE
639 North Larchmont Boulevard
Los Angeles, CA 90004
323-580-6383

300 South Sante Fe Avenue
Los Angeles, CA 90013
213-929-5580

512 Rose Avenue
Venice, CA 90291
424-231-8000
cafegratitude.com

HONEY HI
1620 West Sunset Boulevard
Los Angeles, CA 90026
213-221-7810
honeyhi.co

BAROO
5706 Santa Monica Boulevard
Los Angeles, CA 90038
323-929-9288
baroola.strikingly.com

INAKA
131 South La Brea
Avenue
Los Angeles, CA
90036
323-936-9353
inakanaturalfoods.com

MOON JUICE
8463-3 Melrose Place
323-852-3414
2829 Sunset
Boulevard
213-908-5407
507 Rose Avenue
310-399-2929
moonjuice.com

KIPPY'S
245 Main Street #3D
Venice, CA 90291
424-387-8765
kippysicecream.com

BACKYARD BOWLS
8303 Beverly
Boulevard
Los Angeles, CA
90048

323-746-5404
backyardbowls.com

BOTANICA
1620 Silverlake
Boulevard
Los Angeles, CA
90026
323-522-6106
botanicarestaurant.com

EATING IN: SHOPS AND MARKETS

These are the spots that keep our fridges and cupboards stocked with the building blocks of a High Vibrational lifestyle. All in good taste.

NEW YORK CITY

INTEGRAL YOGA
227 West 13th Street
New York, NY 10011
212-929-0585
iyiny.org/integralyoga
-shop

HIGH VIBE
138 East 3rd Street
New York, NY 10009
800-554-6645
highvibe.com

LIFETHYME
410 Sixth Avenue
New York, NY 10011
212-420-1600
lifethymemarket.com

EATALY
200 Fifth Avenue
New York, NY 10010
212-229-2560
eataly.com

PERELANDRA
175 Remsen Street
Brooklyn, NY 11201
718-855-6068
perelandranatural.com

GREENMARKET NYC
East 17th Street &
Union Square West
New York, NY 10038
grownyc.org
/greenmarket

**LIVE LIVE &
ORGANIC**
261 East 10th Street
New York, NY 10009
212-505-5504
live-live.com

DR-COW
93 South 6th Street
Brooklyn, NY 11249
718-496-7212
dr-cow.com

DIMES MARKET
143 Division Street
New York, NY
10002
646-870-5113
dimesnyc.com/market

FORAGERS
300 West 22nd
Street
New York, NY 10011
212-243-8883
foragersmarket.com

BACK TO THE LAND
142 7th Avenue
Brooklyn, NY 11215
718-768-5654
backtothelandnatural
foods.com

LOS ANGELES

**SANTA MONICA
FARMER'S MARKET**
2640 Main Street
Santa Monica, CA
90401
310-458-8411
smgov.net/portals
/farmersmarket/

EREWHON
585 Venice Boulevard
Venice, CA 90291
323-937-0777
erewhonmarket.com

COOKBOOK
1549 Echo Park
Avenue
Los Angeles, CA
90026
213-250-1900
cookbookla.com

BOTANICA
1620 Silverlake
Boulevard
Los Angeles, CA
90026
323-522-6106
botanicarestaurant.com

ONLINE

THRIVE MARKET
thrivemarket.com

KITCHEN TOOLS

NUT MILK BAG
ELAINA LOVE AMAZING NUT MILK BAG
store.purejoyplanet
.com

HIGH-SPEED BLENDER
VITAMIX
vitamix.com

POPCORN MAKER
WHIRLY POP
whirlypopshop.com

STORAGE CONTAINERS
QUATTRO STAGIONI JARS AND BOTTLES
containerstore.com

WECK JARS
williams-sonoma.com

BORMIOLI ROCCO FRIGOVERRE GLASS FOOD STORAGE CONTAINERS
target.com

PYREX GLASS FOOD STORAGE CONTAINERS
target.com

QUADRO LARGE GLASS JUG
crateandbarrel.com

SARAH KERSTEN COVERED BOWLS
sarahkersten.com

HASAMI PORCELAIN LIDDED BOWL
needsupply.com
tortoisegeneral
store.com
trnk-nyc.com

PRODUCE BAGS
ORGANIC MUSLIN PRODUCE BAGS
ecobags.com

KNIVES
TOGIHARU DAMASCUS NAKIRI AND ASSORTED JAPANESE KNIVES
Korin
57 Warren Street
New York, NY 10007
212-587-7021
korin.com

SINGLE SABATIER KNIVES
Great French Knives
Bon Vivant School of Cooking
4925 NE 86th Street
Seattle, WA 98115
206-525-7537
greatfrenchknives.com

GLASS STRAWS
GLASS DHARMA
capbeauty.com

SLICERS
KYOCERA CERAMIC HANDHELD SLICER
surlatable.com

JAPANESE MANDOLIN
williams-sonoma.com
whisknyc.com

JUICERS
BREVILLE JUICER
williams-sonoma.com

DEHYDRATOR
SEDONA DEHYDRATOR
live-live.com

SPIRALIZER
GEFU HANDHELD SPIRALIZER
crateandbarrel.com

PADERNO SPIRALIZER
padernousa.com
crateandbarrel.com

FOOD PROCESSOR
CUISINART FOOD PROCESSOR
crateandbarrel.com

FERMENTATION CROCK
SARAH KERSTEN CERAMIC FERMENTATION CROCK
quitokeeto.com
sarahkersten.com

POTS
CERAMIC JAPANESE STEAMER
quitokeeto.com

STAUB
staubusa.com

AGA
agamarvel.com

SAMBONET
sambonet-shop.com

CRANE
cranecookware.com

PORCELAIN BAKING DISHES
PILLIVUYT
food52.com

APILCO
williams-sonoma.com

WATER FILTERS
WALTER FILTER
capbeauty.com

CUSTOM AIR AND WATER
customairandwater.com

BERKEY
800-350-4170
berkeyfilters.com

CERAMICS
CASSIE GRIFFIN
cassiegriffin.com

ROMY NORTHOVER
capbeauty.com

CLAM LAB
clamlab.com
oldfaithfulshop.com
theprimaryessentials
.com

NATALIE WEINBERGER
natalie-w.com
theprimaryessentials
.com

SARAH KERSTEN
sarahkersten.com
quitokeeto.com
theprimaryessentials
.com

HASAMI PORCELAIN
theprimaryessentials
.com
needsupply.com

HENRY STREET
henrystreetstudio.com

SHINO TAKEDA
shinotakeda.com

BARI ZIPPERSTEIN
bzippyandcompany
.com

CHRISTIANE PERROCHON
christianeperrochon
.com
net-de-vivre.com

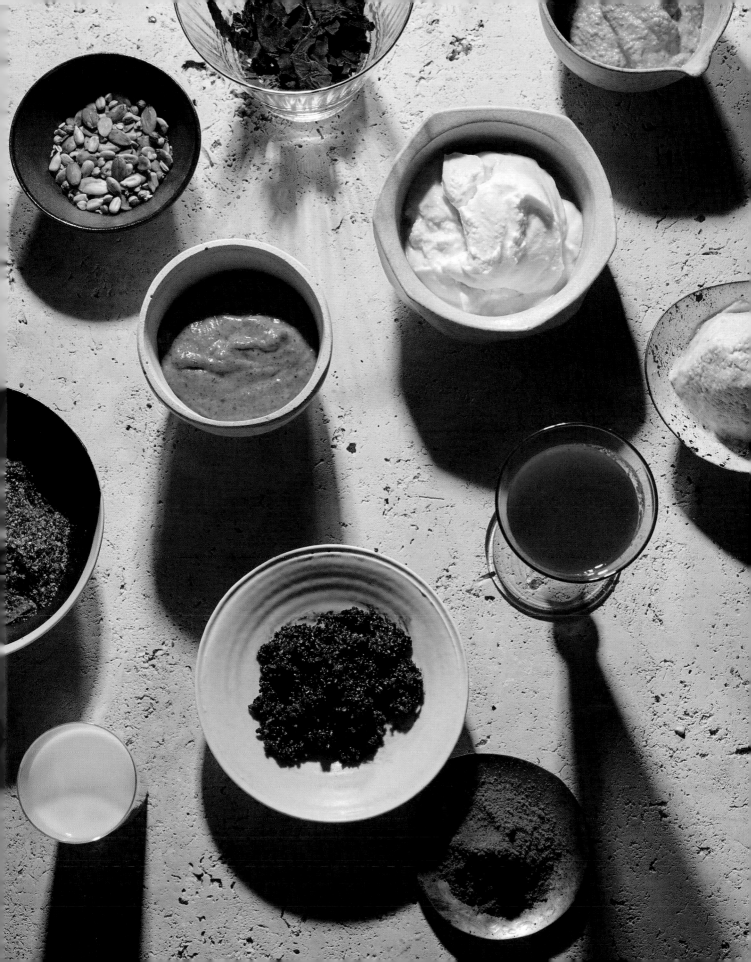

VICTORIA MORRIS
victoriamorrispottery
.com
thefutureperfect.com

COFFEE MAKER
CHEMEX
chemexcoffeemaker
.com
crateandbarrel.com
surlatable.com

*BOWLS AND
BOARDS*
**JASPER CONRAN
WEDGWOOD
"PASTA" BOWL**
wedgwood.com
bloomingdales.com
wayfair.com

**BLACK CREEK
MERCANTILE &
TRADING COMPANY**
blackcreekmt.com

JACOB MAY
jacob-may.com

*SALT, PEPPER
AND SPICE
GRINDERS*
SKEPPSHULT
pleasanthillgrain.com

PEUGEOT
peugeot-saveurs/
en.com
surlatable.com

PERFEX
williams-sonoma.com

PANTRY

TAHINI
SEED + MILL
seedandmill.com
SOOM
soomfoods.com

*GLUTEN-FREE
BREAD*
**GRINDSTONE
BAKERY**
grindstonebakery.com

VEGAN MARIO
veganmario.com

*COCONUT
BUTTER*
**CAP BEAUTY'S THE
COCONUT BUTTER**
capbeauty.com

*PROTEIN
POWDER*
LIVWELL
capbeauty.com

**GREEN ALCHEMY
PROTEIN**
healthforce.com

*ACTIVATED
PUMPKIN,
SUNFLOWER OR
WATERMELON
SEEDS*
GO RAW
goraw.com

*GOLDEN
BERRIES*
THRIVEMARKET.COM

GOJI BERRIES
**DRAGONHERBS
.COM**

*MATCHA
AND TEA*
**CAP BEAUTY'S THE
MATCHA**
capbeauty.com

**CAP BEAUTY'S THE
GENMAICHA**
capbeauty.com

BOTIJA OLIVES
SUNFOOD
vitacost.com
iherb.com
sunfood.com

*ACTIVATED
RAW SEED
CRACKERS*
MOON JUICE
moonjuice.com
capbeauty.com

OLIVE OIL
WONDER VALLEY
capbeauty.com

DRIED BEANS
RANCHO GORDO
ranchogordo.com

*ORGANIC
COFFEE*
CANYON COFFEE
canyoncoffee.co
capbeauty.com

PROBIOTICS
KLAIRE LABS
klaire.com

**ELEMENTAL
WIZDOM**
capbeauty.com

MISO
SOUTH RIVER MISO
southrivermiso.com

HOT SAUCE
**HAWTHORNE
VALLEY**
hawthornevalleyfarm
.org

QUEEN MAJESTY
queenmajestyhotsauce
.com

RANCHO GORDO
ranchogordo.com

*FERMENTED
VEGETABLES*
**HAWTHORNE
VALLEY**
hawthornevalleyfarm
.org

SNACKS
SPLITZ
snacksonsplitz.com

SPROUTIES
gopalshealthfoods
.com

**GOPAL ENERGY
STICKS**
gopalshealthfoods
.com

BJORN QORN
bjornqorn.com

RAWMANTIC BARS
rawmantic-chocolate
.myshopify.com

TUNING IN

MEDITATION

BOB ROTH, THE DAVID LYNCH FOUNDATION
davidlynchfoundation.org

MNDFL
mndflmeditation.com

INSIGHT TIMER
insighttimer.com

SUSIE PEARL
susiepearl.co.uk

PANDIT DASA
panditdasa.com

RA MA INSTITUTE
124 Stanton Street
New York, NY 10002
917-261-6228
or
304 Lincoln Boulevard
Venice, CA 90291
310-664-3700
ramayogainstitute.com

DESIRÉE PAIS
125 Stanton Street
New York, NY 10002
benshen.co

WOOM CENTER
274 Bowery, 2nd Floor
New York, NY 10012
646-678-5092
woomcenter.com

DAVID H. WAGNER
davidhwagner.com

PRACTITIONERS

DANIELA TURLEY
urbanhealingnyc.com

DANA JAMES
foodcoachnyc.com

ROBIN BERZIN
robinberzinmd.com
parsleyhealth.com

LACY PHILLIPS
freeandnative.com

ROSIE REARDON
rosiereardon.com

DANA BALICKI
danabalicki.com

MORGAN YAKUS
morganyakus.com

DANIELLE BEINSTEIN
daniellebeinstein.com

PAULA MALLIS
paulamallis.com

ERICA CHIDI COHEN
thisisloom.com

DAPHNE JAVITCH
doingwell.com

WORKING OUT

SKY TING YOGA
381 Broadway 2nd Floor
New York, NY 10013
212-390-8514
or
55 Chrystie Street, 4th Floor
New York, NY 10002
212-203-5786
skytingyoga.com

DEREK COOK
senseiderek.com

DIANA RILOV
dianarilov.com

TARYN TOOMEY'S THE CLASS
taryntoomey.com

HEATHER LILLESTON
heatherlilleston.com

WOOM CENTER
274 Bowery, 2nd Floor
New York, NY 10012
646-678-5092
woomcenter.com

KULA YOGA
481 Broadway, 3rd Floor
New York, NY 10013
917-472-7499

or
85 North 3rd Street
Brooklyn, NY 11249
347-463-9886
kulayoga.com

NEW YORK PILATES
64 West 3rd Street
New York, NY 10012
and
262 Bowery Street
New York, NY 10013
and
25 Howard Street
New York, NY 10013
212-335-0375
newyorkpilates.com

MODELFIT
212 Bowery
New York, NY 10012
212-219-2044
modelfit.com

LOVE YOGA
2110 Sunset Boulevard
Los Angeles, CA 90025
or
835 Lincoln Boulevard
Venice, CA 90291
323-673-8934
loveyogaspace.com

KAYLA ITSINES
kaylaitsines.com

LAUREN ROXBURGH
laurenroxburgh.com

JIVAMUKTI YOGA
841 Broadway, 2nd Floor
New York, NY 10003
212-353-0214
jivamuktiyoga.com

YOGA AT THE RAVEN
yogaattheraven.com

TRACY ANDERSON
tracyanderson.com

DIÈRY PRUDENT
prudentfitness.com

CLEARING OUT— COLONICS

JEN GONZALEZ
doodyfreegirl.com

GIL JACOBS
347-933-3590

MIKE PERRINE
everydaydetox.org

CLUTTER

HOUSING WORKS
housingworks.org

MATERIALS FOR THE ARTS
mtfa.org

THE REALREAL
therealreal.com

MATERIAL WORLD
materialworld.co

VESTIAIRE COLLECTIVE
vestiairecollective.com

BIG REUSE BROOKLYN
69 9th Street
Gowanus, NY 11215
718-725-8925
bigreuse.org

TEXTILE RECYCLING AT GROWNYC
grownyc.org

THE LIFE CHANGING MAGIC OF TIDYING UP
konmari.com

ACKNOWLEDGMENTS

We'd be nowhere without the engaged, intelligent and forward thinking family that surrounds us. Some are below, all of them are with us.

We consider our team at Rodale to be like family. And we couldn't be more proud to call them our publisher. Their belief in our vision and their longstanding commitment to wellness won us over and we've never looked back. Our editor, Marisa Vigilante, believed in HVB from the get go and let us run wild with our sometimes out-there ideas. Our plant powered designer Rae Ann took our vision, our images and our concept and created a truly beautiful book. Our editorial assistant, Danielle Curtis kept us on track, on time and helped us to further the vision. And of course, the rest of the Rodale crew that brought our book to life, we thank you.

We wouldn't have a book without our visionary agent, Nicole Tourtelot. She believed in it from day one and championed it all over town. This is someone you want on your team. She also liked our homemade chocolate.

Our unofficial artistic director and official photographer, John von Pamer, brought his weird and beautiful eye to every photo and worked relentlessly to make magic.

The inimitable food stylist, Victoria Granof, is a legend for good reason and we've long dreamt of collaborating with her. Manifestation works and our pictures are the better for it. And her hard working and cool assistants, Krystal, Liza and Kristen, kept things moving while keeping us well fed.

Mary Ellen Amato, our brilliant recipe developer, made our dreams come true through her prowess, patience and wit in the kitchen. Her palate and persistence elevated our ideas to what we might humbly say are some of the most delicious and healthy recipes we've tried. And we've tried them all.

Our recipe testing alchemist, Lauren Nicole Schaeffer, tweaked and perfected each recipe allowing you to easily create these magical meals at home.

Graeme Smith, department of dehydration and fermentation, supplied us with our pickles, tart crusts and crackers and gave us something delicious to chew on.

Our beautiful pink haired photo assistant, Sage McAvoy, graced us on the daily with her calm and otherworldly presence.

Our sassy Spanish firefly, Ariadna Pedret, got our props to set with grace, fire and military order. The irreplaceable Dayna Seman helped kick things off.

Thank you to the inspired designers and makers who loaned us their creations to help our book come to life. We're talking to you, Randi Mates of Aesa, Marité Acosta, Lauren of The Primary Essentials and Concrete Cat. Please keep making beauty.

Thank you to Helen and Frank DiPrima, Laurent Morisse, Louise Eastman, Mia McDonald and Tony Dick, Dana and Steve DiPrima, Megan and Rick Foker, Steven Alan, Kelly and Richard Paxton, Barbara Paxton, Kathy and Brian Paxton. Your belief in us through it all has fueled and encouraged us to be our best versions of ourselves. For that we are eternally grateful.

To our CAP family, old and new. You inspire and humble us on the daily. Your hard work, your passion and your commitment to the mission make us proud parents and even prouder to call you friends.

Our customers and clients keep us moving forward. Your belief, curiosity and trust are a true inspiration.

To the creators of the products that line our shelves. We're nothing without you. Thank you for taking this journey with us.

To the aforementioned John von Pamer, this time in the role of my husband. Your engagement, curiosity, constant questioning and all-consuming love make me a better person. And your playlists make me happy too.

To Laurent, Louis and Sally Morisse, I do my best at home and at work to make the world a better place for all of us. I couldn't be more proud to be the wife and mama of our crew.

To all of you out there who believe in the power of plants, rituals and Mother Earth. The best is yet to come.

INDEX

Before launching CAP Beauty, **KERRILYNN PAMER** and **CINDY DIPRIMA MORISSE** were deeply entrenched in the worlds of style, lifestyle, food and design. While working at Martha Stewart Living, they quickly bonded over a shared love of fashion, cooking, interiors and wellness. They founded CAP Beauty in 2014 and live by the motto "Beauty is Wellness." They hope to share the power of natural beauty (and all that it encompasses) with as many as possible. Kerrilynn resides in Los Angeles with her husband, John, and their two rescue Chihuahuas, Beba and Ricardo. Cindy resides in New York City with her husband, Laurent, and their two children, Louis and Sally. They talk on the phone daily.